# Dermatology

An International Journal founded as
'Dermatologische Zeitschrift' by Oskar Lassar (1893–1907)
Continued by Erich Hoffmann (1908–1938), continued as 'Dermatologica' (1939–1991),
by Wilhelm Lutz (1939–1958), Rudolf Schuppli (1959–1985)



**From 2008 on this journal is proud to publish newsletters and papers from the International League of Dermatologic Societies, edited by R.J. Hay and R. Marks**

KARGER

Printed in Switzerland
on acid-free and non-aging
paper (ISO 9706) by
Reinhardt Druck, Basel

Appears 6-weekly:
2 volumes per year
(8 issues)

# Guidelines for Authors

# Dermatology

## Submission

Only original papers written in English should be sent to:

**www.karger.com/drm**

Prof. J.-H. Saurat
S. Karger AG
Editorial Office 'Dermatology'
PO Box
CH–4009 Basel (Switzerland)
Tel. +41 61 306 1356
Fax +41 61 306 1434
E-Mail drm@karger.ch

## Conditions

All manuscripts are subject to editorial review. Manuscripts are received with the explicit understanding that they are not under simultaneous consideration by any other publication. Submission of an article for publication implies transfer of the copyright from the author to the publisher upon acceptance. Accepted papers become the permanent property of 'Dermatology' and may not be reproduced by any means, in whole or in part, without the written consent of the publisher. It is the author's responsibility to obtain permission to reproduce illustrations, tables, etc. from other publications.

## Sections

The journal consists of the following sections:

- Editorials
- Original Papers
- Case and Review (This section contains case reports extended with literature reviews.)
- Case Reports
- Letters to Dermatology

We proudly publish the Newsletter of the International League of Dermatological Societies (ILDS).

## Topics

Please submit papers of the following topics:

- Clinical and Laboratory Studies
- Dermatopathology
- Dermatosurgery and Related Interventional Techniques
- Imaging Techniques
- Evidence-Based Dermatology
- Pharmacology and Treatment

## Conflicts of Interest

Authors are required to disclose any sponsorship or funding arrangements relating to their research and all authors should disclose any possible conflicts of interest. Conflict of interest statements will be published at the end of the article.

## Ethics

Published research must comply with the guidelines for human studies and animal welfare regulations. Authors should state that subjects have given their informed consent and that the study protocol has been approved by the institute's committee on human research. Further, they should also state that animal experiments conform to institutional standards.

## Rapid Communications/Hot Topics

Authors may apply to have their paper treated as a rapid communication. Condition for this is a brief definite report of important results. Final decision whether a paper will be published as a rapid communication will be made by the Editors. A publication time of three months after acceptance is intended.

## Arrangement

Papers should comprise approximately 13 pages including figures, tables and references. For technical details please refer to: **www.karger.com/electronic_submission**.

*Title page:* The first page of each paper should indicate the title, the authors' names, the institute where the work was conducted, and a short title for use as running head.
NB: Authors wishing to preserve the phonetic meaning of diacritics (PubMed reduces diacritics to their root characters) must spell their names accordingly when submitting manuscripts (e.g. Müller should be Mueller).

*Full address:* The exact postal address of the corresponding author complete with postal code must be given at the bottom of the title page. Please also supply phone and fax numbers, as well as e-mail address.

*Key words:* For indexing purposes, a list of 3–10 key words in English is essential for all papers.

*Abstract:* Normally each paper needs an abstract of not more than **150 words.** It should contain the following information: purpose of the study, procedures, results, conclusions and message of the paper.
Abstracts submitted for publication in the section Original Papers should be structured as follows:

| | |
|---|---|
| *Background:* | What is the major problem that prompted the study? |
| *Objective:* | What is the purpose of the study? |
| *Methods:* | How was the study performed? |
| *Results:* | Most important findings? |
| *Conclusion:* | Most important conclusion? |

*Footnotes:* Avoid footnotes. When essential, they are numbered consecutively and typed at the foot of the appropriate page.

*Tables and illustrations:* Tables and illustrations (both numbered in Arabic numerals) should be stored in separate files. Tables require a heading and figures a legend, also prepared on a separate file. When possible, group several illustrations in one block for reproduction (max. size 180 × 223 mm) or provide crop marks. B/w half-tone and color illustrations must have a final resolution of 300 dpi after scaling, line drawings one of 800–1,200 dpi. For further details please refer to the Submission Website at **www.karger.com/drm**.

*Color illustrations:* During the review process, the decision will be made as to which color illustrations of a manuscript can be reproduced free of charge. Authors will be informed of this at the time of acceptance of their paper. Otherwise, these illustrations will be reproduced at the author's expense. Up to 6 color illustrations per page can be integrated into the text at the special price of CHF 800.– per page.

*Anonymity in Case Reports:* Authors should preserve patients' anonymity both in the text and figures, in the case that patients might be identified, authors should obtain his (her) informed consent.

*References:* In the text identify references by Arabic numerals [in square brackets]. Material submitted for publication but not yet accepted should be noted as 'unpublished data' and not be included in the reference list. The list of references should include only those publications which are cited in the text. Avoid using abstracts and posters as references. If necessary list as footnotes in standard reference format, followed by the designation '(abstr.)' or '(poster)'. For posters, add the details of the meeting where presented. Do not alphabetize; number references in the order in which they are first mentioned in the text. The surnames of the authors followed by initials should be given. There should be no punctuation other than a comma to separate the authors. Preferably, please cite all authors. Abbreviate journal names according to the Index Medicus system. (Also see International Committee of Medical Journal Editors: Uniform requirements for manuscripts submitted to biomedical journals. N Engl J Med 1997;336:309–315. **www.icmje.org**).

*Examples*
*(a) Papers published in periodicals:* Chatel JM, Bernard H, Orson FM: Isolation and characterization of two complete Ara h 2 isoforms cDNA. Int Arch Allergy Immunol 2003;131:14–18.
*(b) Papers published only with DOI numbers:* Theoharides TC, Boucher W, Spear K: Serum interleukin-6 reflects disease severity and osteoporosis in mastocytosis patients. Int Arch Allergy Immunol DOI: 10.1159/000063858.
*(c) Monographs:* Matthews DE, Farewell VT: Using and Understanding Medical Statistics, ed 3, revised. Basel, Karger, 1996.
*(d) Edited books:* DuBois RN: Cyclooxygenase-2 and colorectal cancer; in Dannenberg AJ, Dubois RN (eds): COX-2. Prog Exp Tum Res. Basel, Karger, 2003, vol 37, pp 124–137.

*Reference Management Software:* Use of EndNote is recommended for easy management and formatting of citations and reference lists.

## Digital Object Identifier (DOI)

S. Karger Publishers supports DOIs as unique identifiers for articles. A DOI number will be printed on the title page of each article. DOIs can be useful in the future for identifying and citing articles published online without volume or issue information. More information can be found at **www.doi.org**.

KARGER

Fax +41 61 306 12 34
E-Mail karger@karger.ch
www.karger.com



The Guidelines for Authors are available at:
www.karger.com/drm_Guidelines

### Author's Choice™

Karger's Author's Choice service broadens the reach of your article and gives all users worldwide free and full access for reading, downloading and printing at www.karger.com. The option is available for a one-time fee of CHF 3000.–, which is a permissible cost in grant allocation. More information can be found at www.karger.com/authors_choice.

### NIH-Funded Research

The U.S. National Institutes of Health (NIH) mandates under the NIH Public Access Policy that final, peer-reviewed manuscripts appear in its digital database within 12 months of the official publication date. As a service to authors, Karger submits the final version of your article on your behalf to PubMed Central. For those selecting our premium Author's Choice service, we will send your article immediately upon publishing, accelerating the accessibility of your work without the usual embargo. More details on NIH's Public Access Policy is available at http://publicaccess.nih.gov/FAQ.htm#a1

### Self-Archiving

Karger permits authors to archive their pre-prints (i.e. pre-refereeing) or post-prints (i.e. final draft post-refereeing) on their personal or institution's servers, provided the following conditions are met: Articles may not be used for commercial purposes, must be linked to the publisher's version, and must acknowledge the publisher's copyright. Authors selecting Karger's Author's Choice feature, however, are also permitted to archive the final, published version of their article, which includes copyediting and design improvements as well as citation links.

### Page Charges

There are no page charges for papers of 4 or fewer printed pages (including tables, illustrations and references). Each additional complete or partial page is charged to the author at CHF 325.–. The allotted size of a paper is equal to approx. 13 manuscript pages (including tables, illustrations and references).

### Proofs

Unless indicated otherwise, proofs are sent to the first-named author and should be returned with the least possible delay. Alterations made in proofs, other than the correction of printer's errors, are charged to the author. No page proofs are supplied.

### E-pub First

All articles are published electronically ahead of print with a DOI number and are supplemented later with the definite reference of the printed version. The articles become available immediately after the authors' approval to publication, with the added advantage of being citable much earlier than in print. Authors can influence the time of appearance by promptly returning the proofs.

### Reprints

Order forms and a price list are sent with the proofs. Orders submitted after the issue is printed are subject to considerably higher prices.

**2008 Impact factor: 2.227**




KARGER

Fax +41 61 306 12 34
E-Mail karger@karger.ch
www.karger.com




The Guidelines for Authors are available at:
www.karger.com/drm_Guidelines

# Dermatology

## General Information

**ISSN Print Edition:** 1018–8665
**ISSN Online Edition:** 1421–9832

**Journal Homepage:** www.karger.com/drm

**Publication Data:** 'Dermatology' is published 8 times a year. Volumes 220–221, each with 4 issues, appear in 2010.



**Subscription Rates:** Subscriptions run for a full calendar year. Prices are given per year.
*Personal subscription:*

| **Print or Online** | **Print+Online combined** |
|---|---|
| CHF 1239.– | CHF 1329.– |
| EUR 885.– | EUR 949.– |
| USD 1124.00 | USD 1210.00 |

**postage and handling** (added to print and print+online)
CHF 50.40 Europe, CHF 75.60 Overseas
EUR 36.–
USD 71.60

*Institutional subscription:*

| **Print or Online** | **Print+Online combined** |
|---|---|
| CHF 2478.– | CHF 2726.– |
| EUR 1770.– | EUR 1948.– |
| USD 2248.00 | USD 2472.00 |

**postage and handling** (added to print and print+online)
CHF 63.20 Europe, CHF 94.40 Overseas
EUR 44.80
USD 89.60

*Airmail surcharge:* CHF 64.– / USD 60.80
*Discount subscription prices:*
For members of Dermatology Societies.

**Back Volumes and Single Issues:** Information on availability and prices of single print issues and print or electronic back volumes can be obtained from Customer Service at *service@karger.ch.*

**Bibliographic Indices:** This journal is regularly listed in bibliographic services, including *Current Contents®* and PubMed/MEDLINE.

**Photocopying:** This journal has been registered with the Copyright Clearance Center (CCC), as indicated by the code appearing on the first page of each article. For readers in the US, this code signals consent for copying of articles for personal or internal use, or for the personal or internal use of specific clients, provided that the stated fee is paid per copy directly to
Copyright Clearance Center Inc.
222 Rosewood Drive
Danvers, MA 01923 (USA)
A copy of the first page of the article must accompany payment. Consent does not extend to copying for general distribution, for promotion, for creating new works, or for resale. In these cases, specific written permission must be obtained from the copyright owner,
S. Karger AG, P.O. Box
CH–4009 Basel (Switzerland).

**Subscription Orders:**
Orders can be placed at agencies, bookstores, directly with the Publisher or further Karger offices or representatives:

S. Karger AG
Medical and Scientific Publishers
P.O. Box
CH–4009 Basel
Switzerland
(for courier services only:
Allschwilerstrasse 10
CH–4055 Basel)
Tel. +41 61 306 11 11
Fax +41 61 306 12 34
E-Mail karger@karger.ch
www.karger.com

*France:*
Librairie Medi-Sciences Sarl
36, bd de Latour-Maubourg
75007 Paris
France
Tél. +33 1 45 51 42 58
Fax +33 1 45 56 07 80
E-Mail librairie@medi-sciences.fr
www.medi-sciences.fr

*Germany:*
S. Karger GmbH
Postfach
79095 Freiburg
Deutschland
(Hausadresse: Wilhelmstrasse 20 A
79098 Freiburg)
Tel. +49 761 45 20 70
Fax +49 761 45 20 714
E-Post information@karger.de
www.karger.de

*India, Bangladesh, Sri Lanka:*
Panther Publishers Private Ltd.
33, First Main
Koramangala First Block
Bangalore 560 034
India
Tel. +91 80 25505 836
Tel. +91 80 25505 837
Fax +91 80 25505 981
E-Mail panther_publishers@vsnl.com
www.pantherpublishers.com

*Japan:*
Karger Japan, Inc.
Yushima S Bld. 3F
4-2-3, Yushima, Bunkyo-ku
Tokyo 113-0034
Japan
Tel. +81 3 3815 1800
Fax +81 3 3815 1802
E-Mail publisher@karger.jp

*China, Taiwan and Malaysia:*
Karger China
Suite 409, Apollo Building
1440 Central Yan An Road
Shanghai 200040
China
Tel. +86 21 6133 1861
Fax +86 21 6133 1862
E-Mail karger.ray@gmail.com

*South America and Central America:*
Cranbury International LLC
7 Clarendon Ave., Suite 2
Montpelier, VT 05602
USA
Tel. +1 802 223 6565
Fax +1 802 223 6824
E-Mail
eatkin@cranburyinternational.com
www.cranburyinternational.com

*United Kingdom, Ireland:*
S. Karger AG
c/o London Liaison Office
4 Rickett Street
London SW6 1RU
United Kingdom
Tel. +44 20 7386 0500
Fax +44 20 7610 3337
E-Mail uk@karger.ch

*USA:*
S. Karger Publishers, Inc.
26 West Avon Road
P.O. Box 529
Unionville, CT 06085
USA
Toll free: +1 800 828 5479
Tel. +1 860 675 7834
Fax +1 860 675 7302
E-Mail karger@snet.net

**Change of Address:**
Both old and new address should be sent to the subscription source.

KARGER

Fax +41 61 306 12 34
E-Mail karger@karger.ch
www.karger.com



The Journal Home Page is available at:
www.karger.com/drm

Dermatology

# Psoriasis: Looking Deeper into Skin and Nail Disease

Editors
*Jean-Hilaire Saurat,* Geneva
*Kristian Reich,* Hamburg

16 figures, 8 in color, and 15 tables, 2010

KARGER
Basel · Freiburg · Paris · London · New York · Bangalore · Bangkok · Shanghai · Singapore · Tokyo · Sydney

This supplement was sponsored by
Essex Chemie Ltd., a subsidiary of Merck & Co., Inc.

S. Karger
Medical and Scientific Publishers
Basel • Freiburg • Paris • London •
New York • Bangalore • Bangkok •
Shanghai • Singapore • Tokyo • Sydney



Drug Dosage
The authors and the publisher have exerted every effort to ensure that drug selection and dosage set forth in this text are in accord with current recommendations and practice at the time of publication. However, in view of ongoing research, changes in government regulations, and the constant flow of information relating to drug therapy and drug reactions, the reader is urged to check the package insert for each drug for any change in indications and dosage and for added warnings and precautions. This is particularly important when the recommended agent is a new and/or infrequently employed drug.


Printed in Switzerland
on acid-free and non-aging paper (ISO 9706) by
Reinhardt Druck, Basel
ISBN 978–3–8055–9554–4
e-ISBN 978–3–8055–9555–1

KARGER

Fax +41 61 306 12 34
E-Mail karger@karger.ch
www.karger.com

Vol. 221, Suppl. 1, 2010

Dermatology

# Contents



KARGER

Fax +41 61 306 12 34
E-Mail karger@karger.ch
www.karger.com



Access to full text and tables of contents, including tentative ones for forthcoming issues:
www.karger.com/drm_issues

Dermatology

Dermatology 2010;221(suppl 1):1–5
DOI: 10.1159/000316169

Published online: August 9, 2010

# The Burden of Nail Psoriasis: An Introduction

Robert Baran

Nail Disease Center, Cannes, France

**Key Words**
Nail · Psoriasis · Burden of disease

**Abstract**
Nail involvement is an extremely common feature of psoriasis and affects approximately 50% of patients. Despite this, it is an often overlooked feature of the disease, and treatment tends to be focused on clearing the cutaneous component of psoriasis. Clinical manifestations of nail psoriasis are pitting, discolouration, onycholysis and subungual hyperkeratosis as well as nail plate crumbling and splinter haemorrhages. Nail psoriasis is associated with discomfort in many patients and leads to significant functional impairment and psychological stress. The often distressing appearance of affected nails impacts the patient tremendously in both work and social activities. Importantly, 80% of patients with psoriatic arthritis have nail psoriasis. This review discusses the incidence of nail psoriasis and the burden on the patient and illustrates when dermatologists are strategically placed to detect the early signs of more severe disease by promptly diagnosing and managing the nail component of psoriasis.



## Introduction

Psoriasis is a chronic inflammatory skin disease characterised by T-lymphocyte-mediated hyperproliferation of keratinocytes in the skin [1, 2]. Inflammation plays a key role in the pathogenesis of psoriasis. Normally, an immune system response to foreign antigens and subsequent inflammation is short-lived. In psoriasis, however, the immune response is prolonged, leading to sustained inflammation that drives the initiation/exacerbation of the symptoms of psoriasis [3]. Activated inflammatory cells, particularly T cells, and proinflammatory cytokines contribute to the development and proliferation of psoriatic plaques. The most common form of the disease is psoriasis vulgaris, which is characterised by red papulosquamous plaques covered by white or silvery scales. As the nail is a specialised modification of the skin that arises from the epidermis [4], it is not surprising that nail involvement is common in patients with psoriasis.

This supplement will provide a basic overview of the anatomy/pathology of nail disease and include a scientific discussion about why psoriasis with nail involvement is an important matter for the clinical dermatologist to consider due to its impact on patients in both the short and long term. New thinking about the link between the nail and joint illustrates the inflammatory nature of psoriasis and helps us understand that the management of inflammation can influence outcomes. Other sections will highlight the assessment of nail disease and describe critical considerations in the management of both skin and nail disease in the long term. These include current treatment options that address both cutaneous and nail psoriasis and how effective management of psoriasis can lead to the best outcomes. First, we will explore the burden of nail disease and the toll it takes on a patient suffering from the disorder.

KARGER

Fax +41 61 306 12 34
E-Mail karger@karger.ch
www.karger.com


1018–8665/10/2215–0001$26.00/0

Accessible online at:
www.karger.com/drm

Robert Baran, MD
Nail Disease Center
FR–06400 Cannes (France)
Tel. +33 493 339 966, Fax +33 492 988 030
E-Mail baran.r@club-internet.fr

## Incidence

Psoriasis affects 2–3% of the world's population [2]. In its more severe forms, it is extremely distressing for many sufferers [1]. Although skin symptoms are the most common clinical manifestations of psoriasis, concurrent nail involvement is present in between 50% [5] and 56% [6] of patients; in many cases, this involvement causes functional impairment of manual dexterity, pain and psychological stress, placing a significant burden on the patient [1]. In fact, some studies have shown that psoriatic nail lesions affect up to 79% of patients [7, 8]. Indeed, the lifetime incidence of nail involvement in patients with psoriasis has been estimated to be between 80% and 90% [1, 9]. Nail lesions, however, rarely appear as the only clinical symptom of psoriasis [1], as psoriasis limited to the nails occurs in only 1–5% of patients with psoriasis [10].

The clinical signs of nail psoriasis result from the effects of the disease in either the nail bed or the nail matrix (table 1) [11]. Some common clinical signs are pitting, onycholysis, subungual hyperkeratosis, nail bed discolouration, nail plate abnormalities and splinter haemorrhages [1]. Pitting and onycholysis are the most common nail changes, occurring in 68% and 67% of patients, respectively (fig. 1) [1, 7].

**Table 1.** Clinical signs of nail psoriasis [adapted from 11]

| Nail bed and/or hyponychium psoriasis | Nail matrix psoriasis |
|---|---|
| Onycholysis | Pitting |
| Splinter haemorrhages | Transverse grooves |
| Oil drop (salmon patch) discolouration | Trachyonychia |
| Nail bed hyperkeratosis | Leuconychia |
| | Red spots in the lunula |
| | Nail plate thickening |
| | Nail plate crumbling |

## Burden of Nail Psoriasis

Nail involvement in psoriasis impacts the patient in both the short and long term. For many, nail psoriasis leads to significant functional impairment, pain and psychological stress and has a negative impact on social and work activities [11]. The vast majority of psoriasis patients with nail involvement (90%) find the cosmetic appearance of affected nails distressing (fig. 2) [11]. Often, the affected nail plates will thicken and crumble, causing pain and embarrassment and forcing patients to hide their hands and/or feet or shy away from social or business interactions [7, 11, 12]. People with nail psoriasis may have manual dexterity difficulties, including the completion of such common tasks as buttoning clothes and handling small objects. The correlation of decreased social interactions and manual dexterity difficulties may contribute to the higher anxiety and depression scores in patients with severe nail disease. Clinical implications, such as the risk of infection in diseased nails, can also be particularly hindering to social interaction when there is a risk of infection transmission [11]. Even systemic treatment with retinoids (etretinate, acitretin) may be a burden for patients with paronychia, pyogenic granuloma or nail loss [13].

One recent multicentre, cross-sectional, epidemiological study assessed disease severity, health-related quality of life and health care in 1,511 plaque-type psoriasis patients. The assessments were based on data documented by dermatologists during the patients' routine visits, including general patient demographics, Psoriasis Area and Severity Index (PASI), Dermatology Life Quality Index (DLQI) and the 5-dimensional EuroQoL questionnaire. Of these patients, 48.9% suffered from moderate to severe psoriasis and 48.1% had nail involvement [14]. Interestingly, the incidence of nail psoriasis was significantly higher in patients with moderate and severe psoriasis (54.2% and 61.2%, respectively) compared with patients with mild psoriasis (41.3%) (fig. 3). Patients with severe psoriasis (PASI >20) showed reduced health-related quality of life; additionally, these patients had a higher proportion of inability to work, longer periods of lost work and higher proportions of hospitalisation. Among patients with severe psoriasis, only 45.4% had ever been prescribed systemic treatments that might be needed to improve their standard of care [14].

In 2004, a French epidemiological study reviewed the characteristics of patients affected by nail psoriasis. Four thousand surveys were sent to members of the French Association of Psoriasis Patients, with a 33% response rate (n = 1,309). The majority of survey respondents (57.3%) were female, with an average age of 52 years. Approximately 61% of patients with psoriasis had nail involvement, and according to the DLQI, their disease had a high impact on their quality of life, with an average DLQI of 8.3 (SD = 6.5) [15]. Although many patients reported that they had been treated for their psoriasis (64.9%), the vast majority were not satisfied with their treatment (72%). More than one third of patients with nail psoriasis experienced some sort of discomfort due to nail psoriasis, and

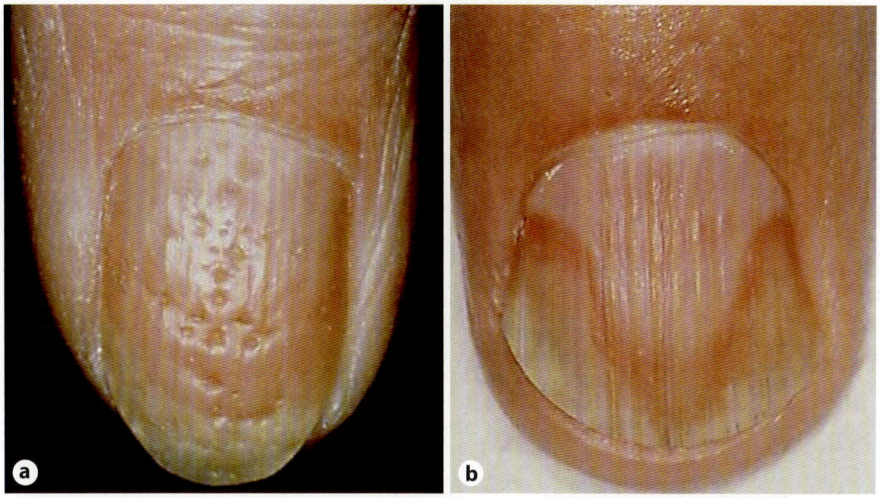


**Fig. 1.** Most common nail changes. **a** Pitting. **b** Onycholysis.

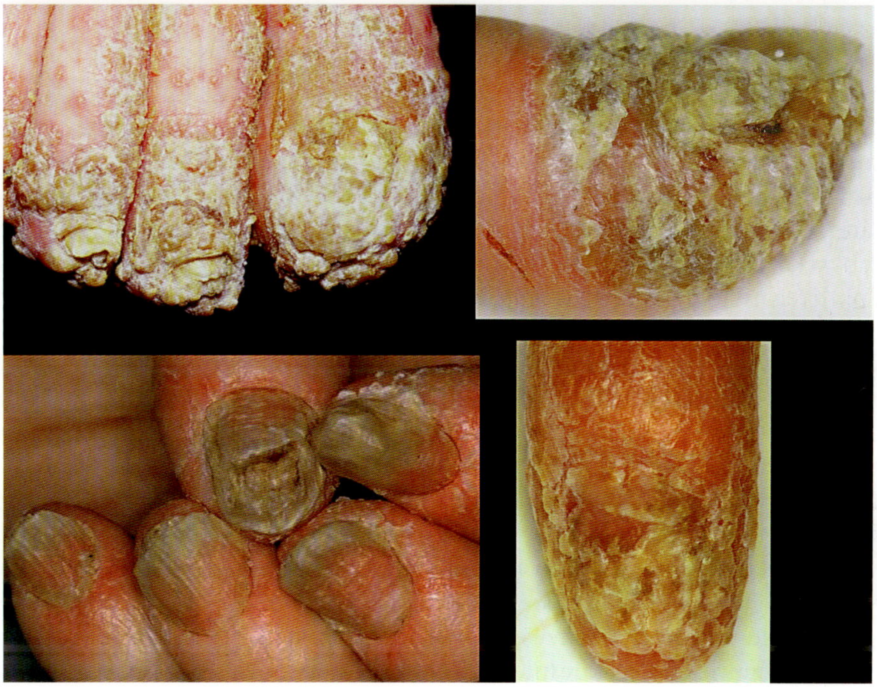

**Fig. 2.** Cosmetic appearance of nail psoriasis.

more than one third suffered considerably from pain and functional discomfort due to nail psoriasis. Approximately 46% of patients considered nail psoriasis to be an aesthetic issue from which they also felt discomfort. In these patients, nail psoriasis had a serious impact on quality of life and the treatments used were not sufficiently effective in nail disease [15].

Little information is available on how severely patients are affected by psoriasis of the nails. de Jong et al. [7] interviewed 1,728 patients with psoriasis via mailed questionnaires and asked about their nail changes and complaints associated with nail involvement. The results indicated that 79.2% of patients had nail psoriasis that clinically manifested most commonly as pitting, deformity, upward lifting, onycholysis and discolouration. Fingernails proved to be more frequently affected than toenails, but both were affected in the majority of patients (62.6%). Approximately 55% of patients had minor complaints and 20.5% had severe problems concerning their nails. Complaints included pain, cosmetic problems and restrictions in daily activity, housekeeping and working. The most concerning aspects of nail psoriasis were the

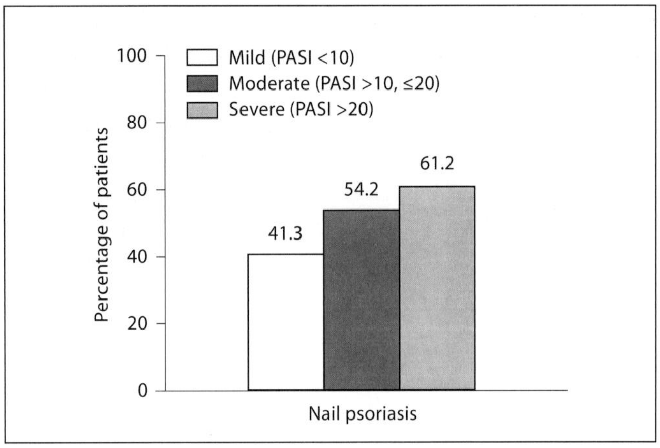


**Fig. 3.** Percentage of patients with nail psoriasis by severity of disease (n = 1,511) [14]. Overall 48.1% were affected by nail psoriasis.

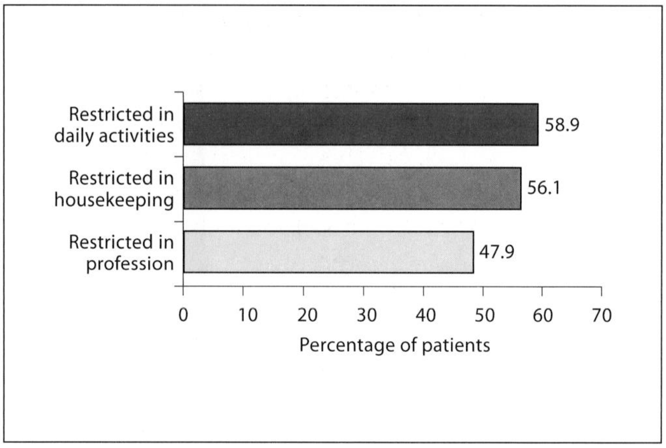


**Fig. 4.** Complaints related to nail psoriasis (n = 1,728) [adapted from 7].

cosmetic problems associated with the disease, as 93.3% of patients were afflicted. Remarkably, 51.8% of patients suffered from pain caused by nail changes and 58.9, 56.1 and 47.9% reported restrictions in their daily activities, housekeeping and/or profession, respectively (fig. 4). With regard to treatment, only 35.4% of patients had used treatment for their nail lesions. Of those patients, only 19.3% showed marked improvement in their disease during treatment, whereas 35% showed little effect and 45.7% showed no improvement at all. This study also found an association between nails and joints, as nail complaints were reported by 52.4% of patients suffering from joint complaints. Of the patients who suffered from joint problems, 85.9% had nail psoriasis [7]. Overall, nail psoriasis seems to greatly affect the psoriatic patient's well-being, and the lack of effective management of nail lesions illustrates a significant need for more effective therapies.

## Beyond the Skin and the Nail

Nail psoriasis not only adds to the burden of disease, but in the long term may also be linked to other aspects of disease. The incidence of nail psoriasis is higher in moderate to severe psoriasis patients and is also associated with a longer duration of disease [7]. Severe nail psoriasis is often correlated with severe skin disease in terms of extent of body surface area involvement and treatment resistance [7]. It is also correlated with enthesitis, polyarticular disease and unremitting and progressive arthritis [16–18]. In fact, nail psoriasis may provide a link in elucidating the pathophysiological variations between skin and joint disease [11]. For example, about 10–20% of patients who have skin psoriasis also have psoriatic arthritis (PsA), a specific condition in which patients have symptoms of both arthritis and psoriasis. Approximately 80% of patients with PsA have affected nails [11]. It is now becoming increasingly clear that psoriasis involves considerably more than its dermatological component and is linked to both nail and joint involvement. The presence of joint or nail symptoms may indicate a more severe form of psoriasis, and this will affect how the disease is managed. It is important, therefore, for dermatologists to be aware of the early symptoms of PsA, particularly in patients with nail psoriasis, in order to avoid progressive joint damage [4, 11, 19, 20]. As dermatologists, we are often in the front line of managing nail involvement in psoriasis and are therefore placed to recognise other symptoms and to provide referral to a rheumatologist as needed.

## Conclusions

Why has our focus on nail psoriasis increased? Despite the recognised burden of nail disease [7], there is a lack of controlled study data related to existing topical, systemic or biologic therapies, and no consistent treatment approach has been advocated [1, 7]. Nail psoriasis is difficult to treat, as nails are slow to heal and conventional treatments are generally difficult to administer and frequently ineffective, with surgery or chemical avulsion sometimes required for refractory cases [21–23]. At times, the management of nail psoriasis is a lengthy, tedious and unsatisfactory process. Systemic drugs such as retinoids, ciclosporin and methotrexate are able to improve both the skin and the nails, but these general immunosuppressants affect the entire immune system and have significant end-organ toxicity. This clinical challenge faced by many dermatologists has recently been addressed with the introduction of the biological response modifiers, which have demonstrated efficacy in both the skin and nail components of psoriasis. Patients who suffer from psoriasis with nail involvement, especially those who are unable to perform normal daily activities owing to related pain or the emotional distress caused by the appearance of affected nails, will benefit from these newer therapies, as targeted biological therapeutics may offer physicians and their patients treatment options that may permit continuous disease control [11].

The identification and effective management of nail involvement in patients with psoriasis are important, as they have both serious and long-term consequences for patients. Physicians are becoming increasingly aware that psoriasis is a disease involving more than just cutaneous symptoms. The link between skin symptoms and both nail and joint signs or symptoms is evident. Consequently, the presence of joint or nail involvement in a patient with psoriasis may indicate a more severe form of the disease and must be taken into consideration when selecting a treatment in order to reduce the pain, functional impairment and emotional distress that may occur during the disease course. By managing the nail involvement effectively, the dermatologist can effectively stop the underlying inflammatory process and potentially limit the progression of disease.

## Conflicts of Interest

Robert Baran serves on scientific advisory boards for Schering Corporation, a subsidiary of Merck & Co., Inc. Editorial support for the development of this publication was provided by Schering Corporation, a subsidiary of Merck & Co., Inc.

## References


1 Jiaravuthisan MM, Dasseville D, Vender RB, Murphy F, Muhn CY: Psoriasis of the nail: anatomy, pathology, clinical presentation, and a review of the literature on therapy. J Am Acad Dermatol 2007;57:1–27.

2 Gudjonsson JE, Karason A, Runardsdottir EH, et al: Distinct clinical differences between HLA-Cw*0602 positive and negative psoriasis patients – an analysis of 1019 HLA-C- and HLA-B-typed patients. J Invest Dermatol 2006;126:740–745.

3 Krueger JG: The immunologic basis for the treatment of psoriasis with new biologic agents. J Am Acad Dermatol 2002;46:1–23.

4 McGonagle D, Tan AL, Benjamin M: The biomechanical link between skin and joint disease in psoriasis and psoriatic arthritis: what every dermatologist needs to know. Ann Rheum Dis 2008;67:1–4.

5 Zaias N: Psoriasis of the nail. A clinical-pathology study. Arch Dermatol 1969;99:567–579.

6 Kaur I, Handa S, Kumar B: Natural history of psoriasis: a study from the Indian subcontinent. J Dermatol 1997;24:230–234.

7 de Jong EMGJ, Seegers BAMPA, Gulinck MK, Boezeman JBM, van de Herkhof PCM: Psoriasis of the nails associated with disability in a large number of patients: results of a recent interview with 1,728 patients. Dermatology 1996;193:300–303.

8 Salomon J, Szepietowski JC, Proniewicz A: Psoriatic nails: a prospective clinical study. J Cutan Med Surg 2003;7:317–321.

9 Samman PD: The Nails in Disease, ed 3. London, William Heinemann Medical, 1978.

10 Van Laborde S, Scher RK: Developments in the treatment of nail psoriasis, melanonychia striata and onychomycosis. Dermatol Clin 2000;18:37–46.

11 Lawry M: Biological therapy and nail psoriasis. Dermatol Ther 2007;20:60–67.

12 Rigopoulos D, Korfitis C, Gregoriou S, Katsambas AD: Infliximab in dermatological treatment beyond psoriasis. Expert Opin Biol Ther 2008;8:123–133.

13 Baran R: Retinoids and the nails. J Dermatol Treat 1990;1:151–154.

14 Augustin M, Krüger K, Radtke MA, Schwippl I, Reich K: Disease severity, quality of life and health care in plaque-type psoriasis: a multicenter cross-sectional study in Germany. Dermatology 2008;216:366–372.

15 Taieb C, Myon E, Voisard JJ, Marin N, Corvest M: Nail psoriasis: epidemiological study in France. Poster presented at the EADV 14th Congress. London, October 2005.

16 Gisondi P, Tinazzi I, El-Dalati G, Gallo M, Biasi D, Barbara LM, Girolomoni G: Lower limb enthesopathy in patients with psoriasis without clinical signs of arthropathy: a hospital-based case-control study. Ann Rheum Dis 2008;67:26–30.

17 Scarpa R, Soscia E, Peluso R, et al: Nail and distal interphalangeal joint in psoriatic arthritis. J Rheumatol 2006;33:1315–1319.

18 Tan AL, Benjamin M, Toumi H, et al: The relationship between the extensor tendon enthesis and the nail in distal interphalangeal joint disease in psoriatic arthritis – a high-resolution MRI and histological study. Rheumatology (Oxford) 2007;46:253–256.

19 Landells I, MacCallum C, Khraishi M: The role of the dermatologist in identification and treatment of the early stages of psoriatic arthritis. Skin Therapy Lett 2008;13:4–8.

20 Williamson L, Dalbeth N, Dockerty JL, Gee BC, Weatherall R, Wordsworth BP: Extended report: nail disease in psoriatic arthritis – clinically important, potentially treatable and often overlooked. Rheumatology (Oxford) 2004;43:790–794.

21 Scher RK: Psoriasis of the nail. Dermatol Clin 1985;3:387–394.

22 De Berker DA: Management of nail psoriasis. Clin Exp Dermatol 2000;25:21–23.

23 Farber E, Nall L: Nail psoriasis. Cutis 1992; 50:174–178.

Dermatology

Dermatology 2010;221(suppl 1):6–14
DOI: 10.1159/000316170

Published online: August 9, 2010

# The Diagnostic and Therapeutic Challenge of Early Psoriatic Arthritis

Paolo Gisondi[a] Ilaria Tinazzi[b] Micol Del Giglio[a] Giampiero Girolomoni[a]

[a]Department of Medicine, Section of Dermatology and Venereology, and [b]Section of Rheumatology, University of Verona, Verona, Italy

**Key Words**
Psoriatic arthritis · Psoriasis · Psoriasis, diagnosis · Psoriasis, therapy

**Abstract**
Psoriasis is a complex disease involving the skin, nails and musculoskeletal structures. Psoriatic arthritis (PsA) affects peripheral joints, entheses, the synovial sheaths of tendons and the axial skeleton. PsA is now recognised as a potentially debilitating disease, with bone erosions and deformities affecting about half of patients and arising early after disease onset. Because PsA usually coincides with or follows the development of psoriasis, dermatologists are in a strategic position to diagnose and manage early PsA. In general, patients with severe psoriasis appear to have a higher risk of arthritis than patients with mild psoriasis. In addition, scalp lesions, nail dystrophy and intergluteal/perianal lesions have been found to be associated with a higher risk of PsA development. The diagnosis of PsA is based primarily on clinical features, and several classification criteria have been developed. Ultrasonography, magnetic resonance imaging and bone scintigraphy, rather than standard radiography, are the most accurate and effective diagnostic imaging approaches for documenting early PsA. The therapeutic strategy for early PsA should be aimed at inducing lasting remission, preventing permanent damage and possibly modifying the natural disease course. 

## Introduction

Psoriasis is a multifaceted disease involving the skin, nails and musculoskeletal structures. Psoriatic arthritis (PsA) affects peripheral joints, entheses, the synovial sheaths of tendons and the axial skeleton [1]. PsA is classified in the spondyloarthritis (SpA) complex together with primary ankylosing spondylitis, reactive arthritis, arthritis associated with inflammatory bowel disease and forms that fail to meet criteria for definite categories, which are designated as undifferentiated SpA [2]. PsA shares with these diseases spinal involvement, extra-articular manifestations and association with the HLA-B27 (human leucocyte antigen-B27) haplotype. Although PsA was formerly considered a mild disease, recent evidence has been gathered indicating that PsA is erosive and deforming in 40–60% of patients, with bone damage arising in the first years after disease onset [3, 4]. Patients with PsA suffer from decreased quality of life (QoL), pain and functional impairment and have a significant increase in mortality compared with the general population [5]. Until a few years ago, the early diagnosis of PsA was not a key concern, especially given the lack of drugs available to alter the disease course. The treatment scenario has completely changed with the introduction of tumour necrosis factor (TNF) blocking agents. The early diagnosis of PsA has now become a challenging topic, as early treatment could avoid irreversible damage and joint deformities [6].

KARGER
Fax +41 61 306 12 34
E-Mail karger@karger.ch
www.karger.com


1018–8665/10/2215–0006$26.00/0

Accessible online at:
www.karger.com/drm

Dr. Paolo Gisondi
Department of Biomedical and Surgical Sciences
Section of Dermatology and Venereology, University of Verona
Piazzale A. Stefani 1, IT–37126 Verona (Italy)
Tel. +39 045 8122 546, Fax +39 045 8027 315, E-Mail paolo.gisondi@univr.it

## Incidence and Prevalence of PsA

The proportion of psoriatic patients developing PsA ranges from 6 to 42% [7, 8]. There are three reasons for the wide variability of these estimates. First, selection bias may be a major problem, as the majority of study populations have been ascertained at referral centres, so patients may predominantly include those with severe disease. Second, the criteria used to identify PsA have been different, with the use of self-reporting methods and/or non-validated definition criteria. Third, the majority of the studies have been cross-sectional and not truly reflective of the evolution of PsA from the time of psoriasis diagnosis to death.

In a recent epidemiological study conducted in Denmark, the prevalence of PsA in the general population was estimated as 0.14% (95% confidence interval [CI]: 0.11%–0.19%) according to the Classification Criteria for Psoriatic Arthritis (CASPAR) [9]. In the United States, the overall age- and sex-adjusted annual incidence of PsA was 7.2 per 100,000 (95% CI: 6.0–8.4), with a higher incidence in men (9.1, 95% CI: 7.1–11.0) than in women (5.4, 95% CI: 4.0–6.9) [10]. More recently, Wilson et al. investigated the cumulative incidence of and clinical predictors for PsA in a cohort of 1,633 subjects with psoriasis followed over a 30-year period [11]. Based on this stable population, the incidence of clinically recognised PsA in psoriasis subjects was 7.5%, which was substantially lower than earlier cross-sectional estimates. PsA usually coincides with or follows the development of psoriasis; it precedes the diagnosis of psoriasis in only 15% of cases. Therefore, dermatologists are in a strategic position to diagnose and manage early PsA or refer the patient to a rheumatologist. PsA can develop at any time, including in childhood, but for most patients, it appears between age 30 and 50.

## Clinical Predictors of PsA in Psoriasis Patients

Although several studies have documented the risk factors for the development and progression of PsA, relatively little is known about the clinical features of psoriasis associated with PsA onset. In general, patients with severe psoriasis appear to have a higher risk of arthritis than patients with mild psoriasis [12]. Oral corticosteroid exposure within 2 years prior to PsA diagnosis, physical trauma and acute life stressors were also found to be associated with the onset of PsA [13]. In particular, biomechanical stress could elicit a Koebner phenomenon on entheses, triggering enthesitis [14]. In contrast, pregnancy has been shown to have a negative association with the onset of PsA [15]. These findings were obtained from relatively small cross-sectional studies or population studies with limited follow-up and a lack of validated PsA diagnostic criteria. In the study by Wilson et al., features of psoriasis that were significantly associated with a higher risk of PsA were scalp lesions, nail dystrophy and intergluteal/perianal lesions [11]. In particular, the risk of PsA was 3.89-fold higher among psoriasis subjects with scalp lesions (hazard ratio [HR]: 3.89; 95% CI: 2.18–6.94) compared with subjects without scalp lesions. Similarly, psoriasis subjects with nail dystrophy were almost 3 times more likely to develop PsA (HR: 2.93; 95% CI: 1.68–5.12) than subjects without nail dystrophy. Previous studies have also suggested that nail dystrophy could be associated with an increased risk of PsA, although not necessarily correlated with disease severity [16, 17]. A recent study by Scarpa et al. suggests that nail involvement is present in almost all cases of PsA, although nail involvement and PsA may not be present at the same time [18]. Indeed, the nail is functionally integrated with the distal phalanx and several distal interphalangeal joint structures, including extensor tendon fibres and the collateral ligaments. The extensor tendon in particular continues from its periostium insertion to envelop the nail root, and the collateral ligaments form a network on the sides of the joint, helping to anchor the nail margins. These findings raise the possibility that nail dystrophy in psoriasis patients could be an indicator of ongoing involvement of the distal phalanx [19]. Clinicians should therefore consider nail dystrophy as highly informative toward predicting the development of PsA. Furthermore, the risk of PsA increased with the number of affected sites; in particular, the risk of PsA in psoriasis subjects with >3 affected sites was 2.24 (95% CI: 1.23–4.08).

Moreover, the demographic, clinical and radiographic characteristics of 40 subjects with PsA who initially presented with psoriasis versus 57 subjects who developed PsA several years after the onset of psoriasis were also examined. PsA subjects who presented concurrently with psoriasis were younger, more likely to be male and more likely to have a family history of psoriasis compared with PsA subjects who developed PsA after psoriasis [11].

## The Clinical Spectrum

The spectrum of joint inflammation in PsA is wide, ranging from axial to peripheral disease. Peripheral arthritis generally presents as inflammatory arthritis, man-

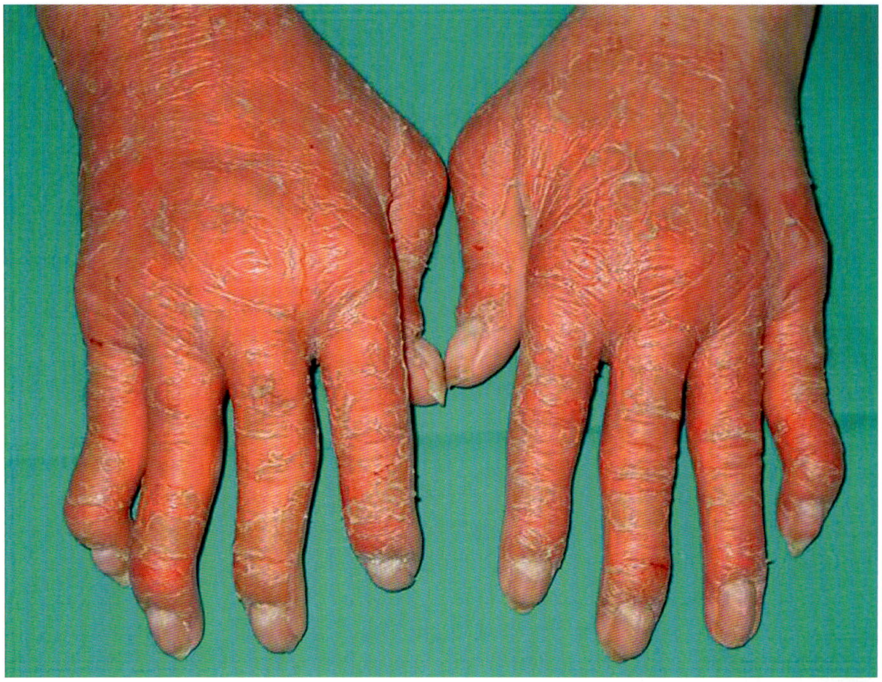

**Fig. 1.** Severe psoriasis of the hands with peripheral arthritis of the distal interphalangeal joints.

ifesting with pain and/or tenderness over the affected joints, with or without joint swelling. The joints of the hands tend to be involved much more frequently than those of the feet, with a ratio of nearly 2:1 (fig. 1). The distribution of affected joints is often in a 'ray' pattern, involving all three joints of an affected digit, whereas other digits are spared. This presentation is in contrast to that of rheumatoid arthritis (RA), in which the joints at the same level tend to be involved, leading to a symmetrical distribution. A typical feature of PsA is reddish/purplish discolouration over the inflamed joint [20]. This is not a common feature of RA, and if a patient has a red joint, infection is suspected. It is sometimes difficult to detect joint effusions in PsA because of the tight capsule. Morning stiffness, a feature of inflammatory arthritis, is detected in about half of patients with PsA. That, taken together with the fact that patients with PsA demonstrate less tenderness than patients with RA [21], has led to underrecognition of PsA and to the misconception that it is a mild condition. Dactylitis, or sausage digit, is also a typical feature of PsA (fig. 2). Dactylitis results from inflammation of both the joints and the tendons, leading to swelling and tenderness of the entire digit. Dactylitis is associated with a higher rate of erosion in the affected digits [22].

Patients with PsA also suffer from tendinitis and enthesitis, which may affect any site, although common locations include the insertion sites of the plantar fascia, the Achilles tendons and ligamentous attachments to the ribs, spine and pelvis. Spondylitis, which includes sacroiliac and apophyseal joint involvement, may present with inflammatory back pain, which usually occurs at rest and immobility but improves with activity and exercise (fig. 3). It is commonly associated with prolonged morning stiffness. Both the sacroiliac changes and the spinal changes are usually asymmetrical in PsA. The SpA of PsA is less severe than that seen in ankylosing spondylitis, as manifested by a lower prevalence of grade 4 sacroiliitis and by better neck and back movement [23].

## Course and Prognosis

Flares and remissions usually characterise the PsA course, which is variable and unpredictable, ranging from mild and non-destructive to severe, debilitating, erosive arthropathy. The severity of the arthritis usually does not correlate with the severity of the skin manifestation. Left untreated, patients with PsA can have persistent inflammation, progressive joint damage, severe physical limitations and disability comparable in severity with that of patients with RA. Indeed, in a cohort of 129 newly diagnosed patients with PsA identified in an early ar-

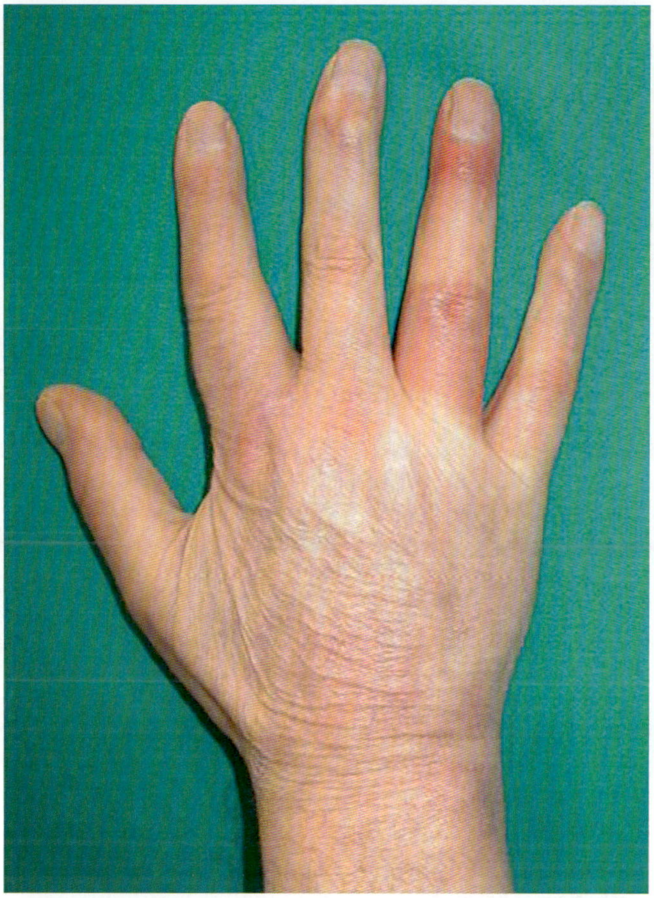

**Fig. 2.** Dactylitis of the fourth digit of the right hand.

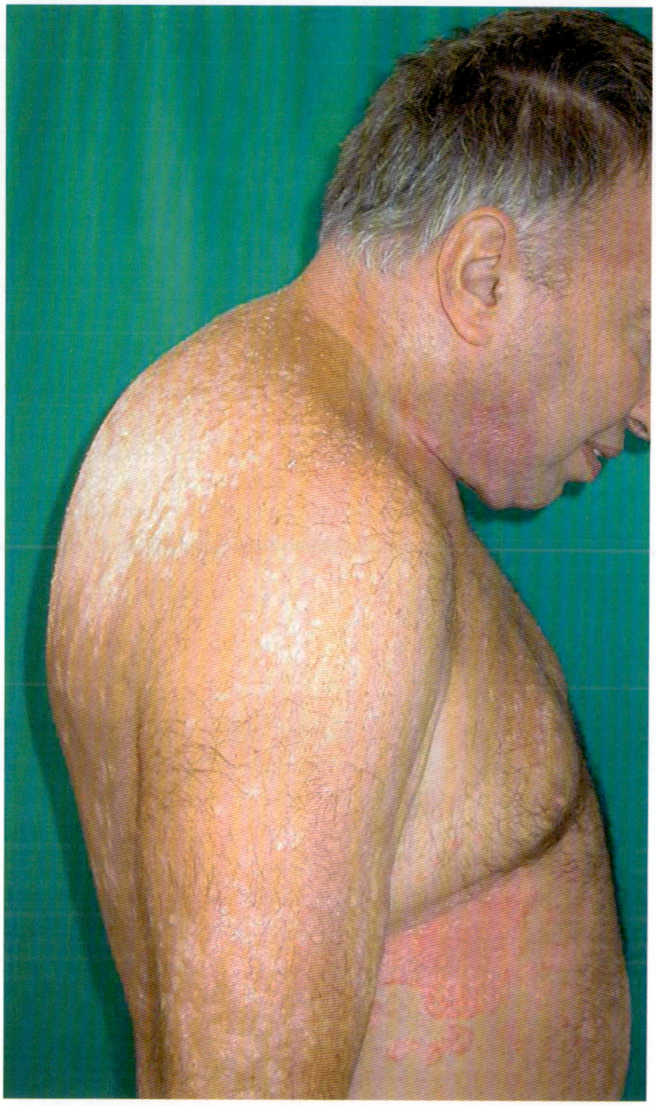

**Fig. 3.** Psoriatic spondylitis with typical cervical involvement.

thritis clinic, the percentage of patients in American College of Rheumatology functional class III/IV (activities of daily living limited to self-care/totally bedridden) was 35% [24]. Progression of radiologic damage by 2 years of disease occurred in 47% of patients, despite clinical improvement with disease-modifying anti-rheumatic drugs (DMARDs). Although it is generally not possible to accurately predict which patients will progress to disabling PsA, one prospective study of 71 patients suggests that polyarticular onset (>5 swollen joints) may predict the appearance of erosive and deforming disease over time, thus necessitating early intervention with more effective therapy [25]. The predictors for progression of both clinical and radiologic damage include tender and swollen joint counts, history of previous damage and elevated erythrocyte sedimentation rate [26, 27].

Recent observations from randomised controlled trials in PsA suggest that C-reactive protein is a risk factor for progression of radiologic damage [28]. Patients with PsA demonstrate reduced QoL, manifested by lower scores on the Medical Outcome Survey Short-Form 36 [29]. Similarly, patients with PsA demonstrate reduced function, as measured by higher Health Assessment Questionnaire (HAQ) scores, which may be as high as those of patients with RA [30]. It has been reported that disease activity is a significant predictor of physical functioning, as measured by the HAQ over the course of PsA, although its effect diminishes over time. This may help to explain any reduced variability in physical functioning in late disease. Joint damage has also been found to be

**Table 1.** Classification criteria for early PsA

| Authors | Reference |
|---|---|
| Moll JM, Wright V | Psoriatic arthritis. Semin Arthritis Rheum 1973;3:55–78. |
| Bennett RM | Psoriatic arthritis; in McCarty DJ (ed): Arthritis and Related Conditions. Philadelphia, Lea & Febiger, 1979, p 645. |
| Vasey FB, Espinoza LR | Psoriatic arthritis; in Calin A (ed): Spondyloarthropathies. Orlando, Grune and Stratton, 1984, pp 151–185. |
| Dougados M et al. | The European Spondylarthropathy Study Group preliminary criteria for the classification of spondylarthropathy. Arthritis Rheum 1991;34:1218–1227. |
| McGonagle D et al. | Psoriatic arthritis: a unified concept twenty years on. Arthritis Rheum 1999;42:1080–1086. |
| Fournié B et al. | Proposed classification criteria of psoriatic arthritis. A preliminary study in 260 patients. Rev Rhum Engl Ed 1999;66:446–456. |
| Taylor WJ et al. | Classification criteria for psoriatic arthritis: development of new criteria from a large international study. Arthritis Rheum 2006;54:2665–2673. |

related to the HAQ score over the course of illness, but there is less evidence to suggest an increasing effect of joint damage on physical functioning with increasing duration of disease [31]. Social and financial implications are also important, both in terms of personal loss and the impact of direct (e.g., medical care) and indirect (e.g., inability to work) costs to society and the patient [32].

There is also evidence of increased mortality among patients with PsA. The standardised mortality ratio was found to be 1.62 in one clinic where patients had been followed prospectively for more than 15 years [33]. Causes of death were mainly cardiovascular diseases. Previously active and severe disease, as manifested by a high erythrocyte sedimentation rate, high medication level and high radiologic damage score at first visit, was predictive of this early mortality [5]. Thus, persistent inflammation in PsA could lead to accelerated atherosclerosis. Early diagnosis and treatment could potentially inhibit the systemic consequences of PsA inflammation, and over the past decade, the mortality risk has improved, possibly related to early and effective therapeutic approaches [34].

### Classification and Diagnostic Criteria

The diagnosis of PsA is based primarily on clinical features. Specific patterns of joint inflammation, together with the absence of rheumatoid factor and the presence of skin and/or nail lesions of psoriasis, aid clinicians in diagnosing PsA. The classification of PsA is an area of debate, as evidenced by the large number of criteria proposed (table 1). Although the five subgroups originally proposed by Moll and Wright in 1973 [35] are frequently used, considerable overlap between these groups is now recognised. The recently developed CASPAR criteria define PsA in the presence of established inflammatory arthritis in patients with clinically evident or a personal or family history of skin and/or nail psoriasis. CASPAR criteria have a specificity of 98.7% and a sensitivity of 91.4% for diagnosing PsA [36]. The CASPAR criteria have been suggested to be useful for the identification of early PsA [37] and both sensitive and specific in a family medicine clinic [38]. However, these criteria are based on the presence of established inflammatory musculoskeletal disease, including peripheral arthritis, spinal disease and enthesitis, and may not be sensitive for identifying initial disease.

To address the issue of early identification of patients with PsA, several screening tools have recently been developed. The first, the Psoriatic Arthritis Questionnaire (PAQ), was developed by Peloso et al. [39]. The PAQ was developed specifically to detect PsA among patients with psoriasis and was found to be useful but not sensitive for identifying nail lesions. Alenius et al. [40] used the PAQ to determine the prevalence of PsA among patients with psoriasis and found that it was not sensitive or specific for that purpose. Husni et al. [41] developed the Psoriatic Arthritis Screening and Evaluation (PASE) questionnaire, which had a sensitivity of 82% and a specificity of 72% for identifying PsA among patients with psoriasis. None of these questionnaires were tested in a wider population, and it is not clear whether they would work in a population of patients not known to have psoriasis. The Toronto Psoriatic Arthritis Screening (ToPAS) questionnaire was developed for use in any patient population [42]. It includes 12 questions as well as pictures of skin and nail lesions. It was tested in a PsA clinic, a psoriasis clinic, a general dermatology clinic, a general rheumatology clinic and a family medicine clinic and was found to have a sensitivity of 86.8% and a specificity of 93%. Although this questionnaire needs to be tested in other settings, it promises to be an excellent screening tool for identifying patients with PsA in a psoriasis population and in the general population. This tool may therefore be used for both clinical detection and epidemiologic studies. In the clinical setting, use of the screening tool may help the dermatologist identify patients who should be referred to a rheumatologist for further assessment. Because the majority of patients present with inflammatory joint disease in the context of skin or nail lesions, use of this tool will facilitate early recognition of PsA. Moreover, a screening tool such as the ToPAS questionnaire can be used in family medicine clinics to identify patients with PsA even before they develop psoriasis, thus allowing the identification of the remaining patients with PsA early in their course.

## Imaging in Early Psoriatic Arthritis

The most appropriate diagnostic imaging approach for use in early PsA has yet to be fully investigated. The utility of ultrasonography or magnetic resonance imaging (MRI) in detecting inflammatory and destructive changes in finger and toe joints, tendons and entheses compared with radiography or clinical assessment in patients with PsA was recently assessed [43]. The study enrolled 15 patients with PsA, 5 patients with RA and 5 healthy control subjects. Each joint of the 2nd to 5th finger (metacarpophalangeal, proximal interphalangeal and distal interphalangeal joints) and the 1st to 5th metatarsophalangeal joints of both hands and feet were assessed for the presence of synovitis, bone erosions and bone proliferations using ultrasonography. The 2nd to 5th flexor and extensor tendons of the fingers were also assessed for insertional changes and tenosynovitis. These changes were assessed in one hand using MRI. Radiographs of both hands and feet were used for bone erosions and proliferations. Results showed that both ultrasonography and MRI were more sensitive for detecting inflammatory and destructive changes compared with radiography or clinical examination. Patients with PsA had more changes in the distal interphalangeal joint than patients with RA. The authors concluded that compared with radiography, ultrasonography and MRI offer the potential for major improvement in the assessment of inflammatory or destructive changes to joints, tendons and entheses in the fingers and toes of patients with PsA.

The value of bone scintigraphy in refining the diagnostic accuracy of enthesoarticular involvement was also demonstrated in a recent study of patients with early PsA [44]. The study included 47 patients with definite PsA (n = 29) or sine psoriasis (n = 18) with articular and/or entheseal involvement for ≤12 weeks. Clinical examination indicated that early PsA was oligoenthesoarthritis in >75% of cases. However, bone scintigraphy revealed that the number of joints and/or entheses with inflammatory involvement was three times greater than that observed on clinical examination. These findings suggest that clinical presentation of oligoenthesoarthritis in early PsA may in fact represent a polyarticular condition in which patients are at increased risk of clinical progression, underscoring the importance of accurate diagnostic imaging in the early disease stage.

## Asymptomatic Rheumatic Involvement in Patients with Psoriasis

We found that entheseal abnormalities can be documented by ultrasonography in clinically asymptomatic psoriatic patients. In particular, the thickness of the lower limb entheses examined and the number of enthesophytes were significantly higher in psoriatic patients than in controls. Bone erosions were not observed in either cases or controls, whereas 6 psoriatic patients had retrocalcaneal bursitis [45]. Similar findings were reported by other authors. In particular, De Filippis et al. found that entheseal abnormalities not detected at clinical examination were present in 25% of 24 patients with psoriasis who underwent ultrasonography [46]. Similarly, Ozcakar et al. found that the mean thickness of the Achilles tendon was significantly higher in psoriatic patients (without clinical signs of enthesitis) than in healthy volunteers [47]. Achilles tendon sonographic abnormalities in 35 of 59 psoriatic patients (59.2%) were also reported by De Simone et al. [48]. However, in this study, 15 patients with PsA (out of 58 patients) were included. Finally, Galluzzo et al. found a high prevalence of involvement of the tendons and entheses of the ankle in clinically asymptomatic PsA patients, suggesting that clinical evaluation underestimates these manifestations [49]. These data con-

**Table 2.** Potential treatments for early PsA

| | |
|---|---|
| Symptomatic agents | corticosteroids (intralesional and systemic), COX-2 inhibitors, non-steroidal anti-inflammatory drugs, sulphasalazine |
| Traditional disease-modifying anti-rheumatic drugs | methotrexate, leflunomide, ciclosporin |
| Biologic agents | adalimumab, etanercept, golimumab, infliximab |

firm that entheseal abnormalities could be quite common in patients with psoriasis without clinical signs of articular involvement and suggest that these findings could be related to entheseal psoriatic inflammation, which is not clinically apparent [14].

## The Challenge of Treating Early Psoriatic Arthritis

The therapeutic strategy for early PsA should be aimed at inducing lasting remission, preventing permanent damage and possibly modifying the natural disease course (table 2). In RA, early diagnosis and early initiation of aggressive therapy have become a primary objective. Studies performed in the last few decades have shown that the early use of DMARDs can prevent the progression of joint damage and functional disability [50]. Although it has been suggested that the early treatment of PsA may also provide better results and protection from disease progression, few studies have been performed to test this hypothesis [51].

Several treatment options are available; however, evidence is lacking regarding the recommended strategy in early PsA. Non-steroidal anti-inflammatory drugs are useful for relieving symptoms but have no effect on joint damage. Local corticosteroid injections may be of great benefit in patients with mono- or oligoarthritis, dactylitis or enthesitis. Although the use of systemic corticosteroids is not supported by evidence, in clinical practice they are commonly used to treat flares of peripheral arthritis. Traditional DMARDs are used in PsA to control the symptomatic manifestations, but there is no evidence that they prevent or significantly decrease the progression rate of structural joint damage. The anti-TNF agents (e.g., etanercept, adalimumab, golimumab, infliximab) reduce the signs and symptoms of inflammation, improve functional status and QoL, maintain long-term remission and inhibit the progression of structural damage in peripheral joints [52–55]. Although treatment with TNF inhibitors can be beneficial, they are expensive and not readily available for all patients. Biologic agents should be considered if patients do not respond to traditional treatment during the first few months. However, in selected cases – such as in patients with active polyarthritis or axial involvement together with extra-articular manifestations (generalised and drug-resistant psoriasis, uveitis or gut involvement) – anti-TNF agents may be the best initial therapeutic approach [56].

## Conclusions

Dermatologists are strongly encouraged to actively look for signs and symptoms of PsA at each visit. If PsA is diagnosed, treatment should be initiated to alleviate signs and symptoms of PsA and prevent structural damage. To date, several unanswered questions remain. Is it possible to define a 'window of opportunity' in the treatment of early PsA? If this is the case, can early treatment with anti-TNF agents be cost-effective? Since anti-TNF agents have the potential to improve the pathophysiology of both skin and joints and to retard disease progression, could their early administration change the clinical picture and, eventually, the epidemiology of PsA by preventing its development in patients who only have psoriasis? How long should treatment be maintained when symptoms have disappeared? Can early treatment of PsA (and psoriasis) with certain drugs alter the natural course of the disease? These questions and many others must be answered.

## Conflicts of Interest

Paolo Gisondi has received lecture fees from Merck-Serono, Wyeth and Schering Corporation, a subsidiary of Merck & Co., Inc. Giampiero Girolomoni has received lecture and consultation fees from Merck-Serono, Wyeth and Schering Corporation, a subsidiary of Merck & Co., Inc., Centocor, Abbott, Janssen-Cilag, Astellas and UCB Pharma. This work was supported by the Ministero della Salute and the Ministero dell'Istruzione, Università e Ricerca Scientifica (Programmi di Ricerca Scientifica di Rilevante Interesse Nazionale).

## References


1 Gladman DD: Psoriatic arthritis; in Harris ED Jr, Budd RC, Firestein GS, et al (eds): Kelley's Textbook of Rheumatology, ed 7. Philadelphia, Elsevier Saunders, 2005, vol 2, pp 1155–1164.

2 Dougados M, van der Linden S, Juhlin R, et al: The European Spondylarthropathy Study Group preliminary criteria for the classification of spondylarthropathy. Arthritis Rheum 1991;34:1218–1227.

3 McHugh NJ, Balachrishnan C, Jones SM: Progression of peripheral joint disease in psoriatic arthritis: a 5-yr prospective study. Rheumatology (Oxford) 2003;42:778–783.

4 Gladman DD, Stafford-Brady F, Chang CH, Lewandowski K, Russell ML: Longitudinal study of clinical and radiological progression in psoriatic arthritis. J Rheumatol 1990; 17:809–812.

5 Gladman DD, Farewell VT, Wong K, Husted J: Mortality studies in psoriatic arthritis: results from a single outpatient center. Prognostic indicators for death. Arthritis Rheum 1998;41:1103–1110.

6 Olivieri I, D'Angelo S, Padula A, Palazzi C: The challenge of early diagnosis of psoriatic arthritis. J Rheumatol 2008;35:3–5.

7 Wilson FC, Icen M, Crowson CS, McEvoy MT, Gabriel SE, Kremers HM: Time trends in epidemiology and characteristics of psoriatic arthritis over 3 decades: a population-based study. J Rheumatol 2009;36:361–367.

8 Gisondi P, Girolomoni G, Sampogna F, Tabolli S, Abeni D: Prevalence of psoriatic arthritis and joint complaints in a large population of Italian patients hospitalised for psoriasis. Eur J Dermatol 2005;15:279–283.

9 Pedersen OB, Svendsen AJ, Ejstrup L, Skytthe A, Junker P: The occurrence of psoriatic arthritis in Denmark. Ann Rheum Dis 2008; 67:1422–1426.

10 Shbeeb M, Uramoto KM, Gibson LE, O'Fallon WM, Gabriel SE: The epidemiology of psoriatic arthritis in Olmsted County, Minnesota, USA, 1982–1991. J Rheumatol 2000;27:1247–1250.

11 Wilson FC, Icen M, Crowson S, McEvoy MT, Gabriel SE, Kremers HM: Incidence and clinical predictors of psoriatic arthritis in patients with psoriasis: a population-based study. Arthritis Rheum 2009;61:233–239.

12 Gelfand JM, Gladman DD, Mease PJ, et al: Epidemiology of psoriatic arthritis in the population of the United States. J Am Acad Dermatol 2005;53:573.

13 Pattison EJ, Harrison BJ, Griffiths CE, Silman AJ, Bruce IN: Environmental risk factors for the development of psoriatic arthritis: results from a case control study. Ann Rheum Dis 2008;67:672–676.

14 McGonagle D, Tan AL, Benjamin M: The biomechanical link between skin and joint disease in psoriasis and psoriatic arthritis: what every dermatologist needs to know. Ann Rheum Dis 2008;67:1–4.

15 McHugh NJ, Laurent MR: The effect of pregnancy on the onset of psoriatic arthritis. Br J Rheumatol 1989;28:50–52.

16 Scarpa R, Del Puente A, di Girolamo C, della Valle G, Lubrano E, Oriente P: Interplay between environmental factors, articular involvement, and HLA-B27 in patients with psoriatic arthritis. Ann Rheum Dis 1992;51: 78–79.

17 Serarslan G, Guler H, Karazincir S: The relationship between nail and distal phalangeal bone involvement severity in patients with psoriasis. Clin Rheumatol 2007;26:1245–1247.

18 Scarpa R, Soscia E, Peluso R, et al: Nail and distal interphalangeal joint in psoriatic arthritis. J Rheumatol 2006;33:1315–1319.

19 McGonagle D, Tan AL, Benjamin M: The nail as a musculoskeletal appendage – implications for an improved understanding of the link between psoriasis and arthritis. Dermatology 2009;218:97–102.

20 Jajic I: Blue coloured skin in psoriatic arthritis. Clin Exp Rheumatol 2001;19:478.

21 Buskila D, Langevitz P, Gladman DD, Urowitz S, Smythe H: Patients with rheumatoid arthritis are more tender than those with psoriatic arthritis. J Rheumatol 1992;19: 1115–1119.

22 Brockbank JE, Stein M, Schentag CT, Gladman DD: Dactylitis in psoriatic arthritis: a marker for disease severity? Ann Rheum Dis 2005;64:188–190.

23 Gladman DD, Brubacher B, Buskila D, Langevitz P, Farewell VT: Differences in the expression of spondyloarthropathy: a comparison between ankylosing spondylitis and psoriatic arthritis. Genetic and gender effects. Clin Invest Med 1993;16:1–7.

24 Kane D, Stafford L, Bresniham B, Fitzgerald O: A prospective, clinical and radiological study of early psoriatic arthritis: an early synovitis clinic experience. Rheumatology (Oxford) 2003;42:1460–1468.

25 Queiro-Silva R, Torre-Alonso JC, Tinturé-Eguren T, López-Lagunas I: A polyarticular onset predicts erosive and deforming disease in psoriatic arthritis. Ann Rheum Dis 2003; 62:68–70.

26 Bond SJ, Farewell VT, Schentag CT, Gladman DD: Predictors for radiological damage in psoriatic arthritis. Results from a single centre. Ann Rheum Dis 2007;66:370–376.

27 Kavanaugh A, Antoni CE, Krueger GG, et al: Infliximab treatment dissociates the effect of CRP on radiographic progression in patients with psoriatic arthritis. Ann Rheum Dis 2007;66(suppl II):417.

28 Gladman D, Mease PJ, Choy EH, et al: Analysis of risk factors for radiographic progression in psoriatic arthritis (PsA): subanalysis of ADEPT. Arthritis Rheum 2007;56(suppl 9):S257.

29 Husted J, Gladman DD, Long JA, Farewell VT, Cook R: Validating the SF-36 health questionnaire in patients with psoriatic arthritis. J Rheumatol 1997;24:511–517.

30 Sokoll KB, Helliwell PS: Comparison of disability and quality of life in rheumatoid and psoriatic arthritis. J Rheumatol 2001;28: 1842–1846.

31 Husted JA, Tom BD, Farewell VT, Schentag CT, Gladman DD: A longitudinal study of the effect of disease activity and clinical damage on physical function over the course of psoriatic arthritis: does the effect change over time? Arthritis Rheum 2007;56:840–849.

32 Olivieri I, de Portu S, Salvarani C, et al: The psoriatic arthritis cost evaluation study: a cost-of-illness study on tumour necrosis factor inhibitors in psoriatic arthritis patients with inadequate response to conventional therapy. PACE working group. Rheumatology (Oxford) 2008;47:1664–1670.

33 Wong K, Gladman DD, Husted J, Long J, Farewell VT: Mortality studies in psoriatic arthritis. Results from a single centre. I. Risk and causes of death. Arthritis Rheum 1997; 40:1868–1872.

34 Ali Y, Tom BDM, Schentag CT, Farewell VT, Gladman DD: Improved survival in psoriatic arthritis (PsA) with calendar time. Arthritis Rheum 2007;56:2708–2714.

35 Moll JM, Wright V: Psoriatic arthritis. Semin Arthritis Rheum 1973;3:55–78.

36 Taylor WJ, Gladman DD, Helliwell PS, et al: Classification criteria for psoriatic arthritis: development of new criteria from a large international study. Arthritis Rheum 2006;54: 2665–2673.

37 Chandran V, Schentag CT, Gladman DD: Sensitivity of the Classification of Psoriatic Arthritis (CASPAR) criteria in early psoriatic arthritis. Arthritis Rheum 2007;57: 1560–1563.

38 Chandran V, Schentag CT, Gladman DD: Are the CASPAR criteria for psoriatic arthritis accurate when applied to patients attending a family practice clinic? Arthritis Rheum 2006;54:4091.

39 Peloso PM, Behl M, Hull P, Reeder B: The psoriasis & arthritis questionnaire (PAQ) in detection of arthritis among patients with psoriasis. Arthritis Rheum 1997;40(suppl 9): S64.

40 Alenius GM, Stenberg B, Stenlund H, Lundblad M, Dahlqvist SR: Inflammatory joint manifestations are prevalent in psoriasis: prevalence study of joint and axial involvement in psoriatic patients, and evaluation of psoriatic and arthritic questionnaire. J Rheumatol 2002;29:2577–2582.

41 Husni ME, Meyer KH, Cohen DS, Mody E, Qureshi AA: The PASE questionnaire: pilot-testing a psoriatic arthritis screening and evaluation tool. J Am Acad Dermatol 2007; 57:581–587.

42 Gladman DD, Schentag CT, Tom BD, et al: Development and initial validation of a screening questionnaire for psoriatic arthritis: the Toronto Psoriatic Arthritis Screen (ToPAS). Ann Rheum Dis 2009;68:497–501.

43 Wiell C, Szkudlarek M, Hasselquist M, et al: Ultrasonography, magnetic resonance imaging, radiography, and clinical assessment of inflammatory and destructive changes in fingers and toes of patients with psoriatic arthritis. Arthritis Res Ther 2007;9:R119.

44 Scarpa R, Cuocolo A, Peluso R, et al: Early psoriatic arthritis: the clinical spectrum. J Rheumatol 2008;35:137–141.

45 Gisondi P, Tinazzi I, El-Dalati G, et al: Lower limb enthesopathy in patients with psoriasis without clinical signs of arthropathy: a hospital-based case-control study. Ann Rheum Dis 2008;67:26–30.

46 De Filippis LG, Caliri A, Lo Gullo R, et al: Ultrasonography in the early diagnosis of psoriasis-associated enthesopathy. Int J Tissue React 2005;27:159–162.

47 Ozcakar L, Cetin A, Inanici F, Kaymak B, Gurer CK, Kolemen F: Ultrasonographical evaluation of the Achilles' tendon in psoriasis patients. Int J Dermatol 2005;44:930–932.

48 De Simone C, Guerriero C, Giampetruzzi AR, Costantini M, Di Gregorio F, Amerio P: Achilles tendinitis in psoriasis: clinical and sonographic findings. J Am Acad Dermatol 2003;49:217–222.

49 Galluzzo E, Lischi DM, Taglione E, et al: Sonographic analysis of the ankle in patients with psoriatic arthritis. Scand J Rheumatol 2000;29:52–55.

50 Emery P: Evidence supporting the benefit of early intervention in rheumatoid arthritis. J Rheumatol 2002;66(suppl):3–8.

51 Scarpa R, Peluso R, Atteno M, et al: The effectiveness of a traditional therapeutical approach in early psoriatic arthritis: results of a pilot randomised 6-month trial with methotrexate. Clin Rheumatol 2008;27:823–826.

52 Mease PJ, Kivitz AJ, Burch FX, et al: Etanercept treatment of psoriatic arthritis: safety, efficacy, and effect on disease progression. Arthritis Rheum 2004;50:2264–2272.

53 Kavanaugh A, Antoni CE, Gladman D, et al: The Infliximab Multinational Psoriatic Arthritis Controlled Trial (IMPACT): results of radiographic analyses after 1 year. Ann Rheum Dis 2006;65:1038–1043.

54 Mease PJ, Gladman DD, Ritchlin CT, et al: Adalimumab for the treatment of patients with moderately to severely active psoriatic arthritis: results of a double-blind, randomized, placebo-controlled trial. Arthritis Rheum 2005;52:3279–3289.

55 Kavanaugh A, McInnes I, Mease P, et al: Golimumab, a new human tumor necrosis factor alpha antibody, administered every four weeks as a subcutaneous injection in psoriatic arthritis: twenty-four-week efficacy and safety results of a randomized, placebo-controlled study. Arthritis Rheum 2009;60:976–986.

56 Kavanaugh AF, Ritchlin CT; GRAPPA Treatment Guideline Committee: Systematic review of treatments for psoriatic arthritis: an evidence based approach and basis for treatment guidelines. J Rheumatol 2006;33:1417–1421.

Dermatology

Dermatology 2010;221(suppl 1):15–22
DOI: 10.1159/000316171

Published online: August 9, 2010

# Nailing down the Genetic and Immunological Basis for Psoriatic Disease

Dennis McGonagle[a] Natalia Palmou Fontana[c] Ai Lyn Tan[a] Michael Benjamin[b]

[a]Section of Musculoskeletal Disease, Leeds Institute of Molecular Medicine, University of Leeds and Chapel Allerton Hospital, Leeds, and [b]School of Biosciences, Cardiff University, Cardiff, UK; [c]Rheumatology Department, Complejo Hospitalario Universitario A Coruña, La Coruña, Spain

**Key Words**

Psoriasis · Nail psoriasis · Nail and joint · HLA-Cw6 · Pathophysiology

**Abstract**

Psoriatic disease encompassing skin, joint and nail involvement is largely viewed as autoimmune – a finding supported by data from animal models, the human leucocyte antigen (HLA)-Cw6 disease association in man, T-lymphocyte infiltration in lesional skin and the favourable skin response to T-cell-directed therapies. However, this immunopathogenetic model only applies to the skin, as recent studies failed to demonstrate a HLA-Cw6 association with the nails or joints. Furthermore, the nails and joints are intimately associated with inflammation at points of ligament or tendon insertion (i.e., enthesitis), so it is now appreciated that both of these sites also share a common microanatomical basis. Moreover, inflammation at insertion sites and nails does not appear to be associated with a particular antigenic territory but is quite diffuse in nature. This suggests that an aberrant response to tissue stressing of the integrated nail-joint apparatus, rather than autoimmunity, is driving the inflammatory process. Therefore, HLA-Cw6-associated type 1 psoriasis is more closely linked to autoimmunity, whereas nail and joint disease may be linked to tissue-specific factors, including tissue biomechanical stressing and microtrauma, that lead to activation of aberrant innate immune responses. These observations that stem from nail disease point toward a relative differential involvement of adaptive and innate immunity in the psoriatic disease spectrum and offer a fresh perspective on the pathophysiology of psoriatic disease and how it can be classified along the immunological disease continuum of self-directed inflammation.



## Introduction

From the original description of the association between psoriasis and psoriatic arthritis (PsA) more than 50 years ago, it became immediately evident that the link between joint and nail disease was much more striking than that between skin and nail disease [1, 2]. This is rather surprising, given that nails are epidermal derivatives. However, a joint-nail relationship has been repeatedly described as a feature of PsA, and it is therefore curious that few dermatologists have explored the possibility of anatomical links between the nail and the distal interphalangeal (DIP) joint.

In recent years, the shared and overlapping features of skin and joint disease have led to the proposal that we should consider skin-, nail- and joint-related involvement that is associated with psoriasis under the guise of psori-

KARGER

Fax +41 61 306 12 34
E-Mail karger@karger.ch
www.karger.com


1018–8665/10/2215–0015$26.00/0

Accessible online at:
www.karger.com/drm

Prof. Dennis McGonagle
Section of Musculoskeletal Disease
Leeds Institute of Molecular Medicine, Chapel Allerton Hospital
Chapeltown Road, Leeds LS7 4SA (UK)
Tel. +44 113 3924 747, Fax +44 113 3924 991, E-Mail d.g.mcgonagle@leeds.ac.uk

atic disease [3]. Nail involvement represents an important subset of psoriasis or PsA-related disease, and nail disease has been difficult to treat effectively [4]. The purpose of this article is to synthesise the emerging microanatomical and genetic data on nail involvement in psoriatic disease to show how these data offer new perspectives on psoriatic disease pathophysiology.

## Anatomy of the Nail, Including Skeletal Appendage Integration

The nails are plates of hard keratin covering the dorsal surface of the distal phalanx of each finger or toe. Their named parts are shown in figure 1 and are briefly explained below. For more comprehensive accounts, the reader is referred to the literature [5–7]. The visible region of each nail is the nail plate, which lies on an epithelium that represents a modified deep region of the epidermis (the nail bed). The plate itself is the counterpart of the stratum corneum, although keratohyalin granules are not involved in its formation [6]. The nail plate is bounded at its base and sides by proximal and lateral nail grooves. Much of a healthy nail plate is pink and semi-translucent, revealing the underlying blood vessels. However, the proximal part of the nail plate (the lunula) is opaque and white. The lunula consists of newly formed keratin and is overlapped by the stratum corneum of the proximal nail fold, which forms an eponychium or cuticle. There is a further reflection of stratum corneum under the distal free edge of the nail plate (the hyponychium). The proximal part of the nail bed acts as a nail matrix, which is responsible for producing the nail plate itself. The thickness of the nail plate reflects the proximal-distal length of the matrix [5, 6]. The lunula is the distal part of this matrix.

As it grows, the nail plate slides horizontally over the nail bed while managing to maintain continuous attachment to it. As with the epidermis elsewhere, the surface area of contact between the nail bed and the underlying dermis is greatly increased. However, in the nail bed, the underlying dermis knits into the epithelium as a series of very deep longitudinal ridges, rather than as dermal papillae in the neighbouring matrix. The ridges are tallest toward the free end of the nail and become shorter and more numerous (via splitting) as the lunula is approached [8]. As discussed later, such anatomical variations could be relevant to a better understanding of psoriatic nail changes such as subungual hyperkeratosis and onycholysis.

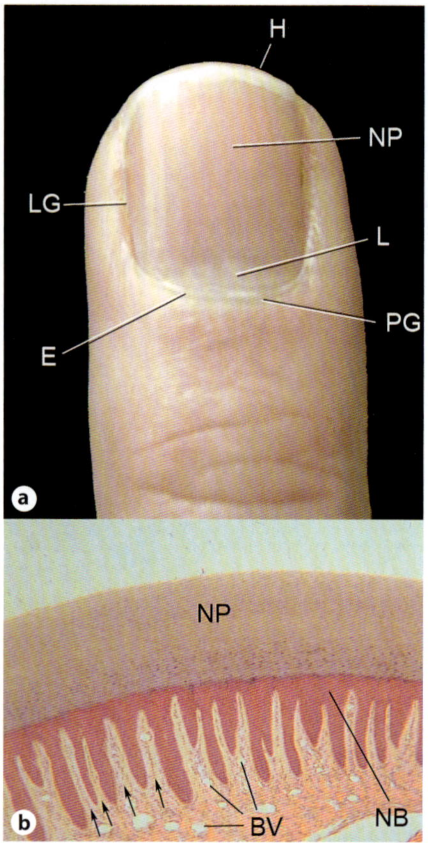


**Fig. 1. a** Parts of the nail. The nail plate (NP) rests on the nail bed (not visible) and has a proximal opaque, whitish semilunar region called the lunula (L). It is bounded at its base and sides by the proximal (PG) and lateral (LG) nail grooves. A fold of stratum corneum (the eponychium, E) overlaps the lunula proximally, and a further reflection of stratum corneum (the hyponychium, H) underlies the free distal edge of the nail plate. **b** A transverse histological section (stained with haematoxylin and eosin) through a nail plate showing the nail plate itself (NP) and the deep longitudinal furrows (arrows) that knit the nail bed (NB) to the underlying dermis like an elaborate series of tongue-and-groove joints. Numerous thin-walled blood vessels (BV) are evident in the dermis itself. These deep ridges are characteristic of the nail plate but not the matrix. This is interesting, since they correspond to the location of splinter haemorrhages.

With respect to the integration of the nail with the local tendon and ligament insertions, collectively termed entheses, several authors have commented that the extensor tendon attaches to the distal phalanx at a site that is very close to the nail matrix. However, we and others have shown that fibres from the tendon actually attach directly to the matrix [9, 10]. We have also drawn attention to a further fascial extension from the enthesis that contributes to a thickening of the periosteum on the adjacent

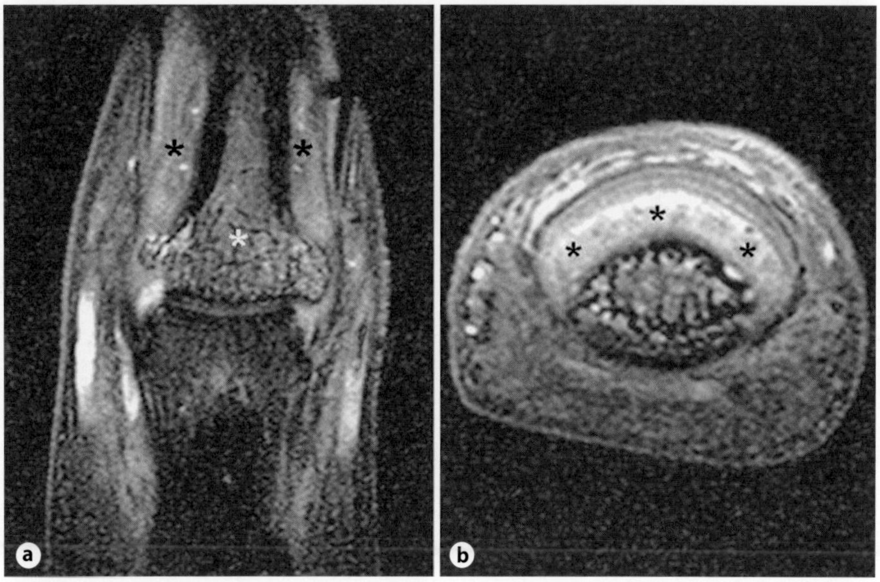

**Fig. 2.** T1-weighted fat-suppressed post-contrast high-resolution MRI of the DIP joint in a 23-year-old man with PsA DIP joint disease in the coronal (**a**) and axial (**b**) planes. These images show the extent of inflammation seen in PsA-related DIP joint disease. Although the enthesis is the epicentre of the inflammatory reaction, there are inflammatory changes extending to involve the adjacent nail-related tissues (black asterisks) and bone (white asterisk). This likely relates to the complex structure of insertions that envelop the nails and to the fact that the nail and enthesis network act as a functional unit.

dorsal surface of the terminal phalanx [5, 10]. As the dermis beneath the nail bed is also anchored to the periosteum, this means that the extensor tendon is both directly and indirectly connected to the nail unit, so the nail plate can be viewed as a skeletal appendage. Importantly, these anatomical studies show that the nail is indirectly attached to the skeleton via the tendon and ligaments' periosteum links [11]. As we shall see later, this bone and enthesis integration is key to an understanding of nail and adjacent joint disease.

## Magnetic Resonance Imaging Studies and Histological Studies in Psoriatic Disease

The resolution of conventional 1.5 T magnetic resonance imaging (MRI) is of limited value for assessing the nail and DIP joint. Consequently, we optimised high-resolution MRI to explore the link between the skin and the DIP joint and noted that polyenthesitis and osteitis were virtually universal in patients with PsA but not in normal individuals [12]. What is particularly significant in the context of the anatomy outlined above is that the PsA-related DIP joint inflammatory reaction was very extensive, enveloped the nail matrix and often extended to the nail bed. Therefore, the inflammatory reaction does not seem to involve a particular tissue or putative autoantigen distribution, but rather the entire joint and nail structure, including bone (fig. 2). These enthesitis-related imaging findings in the DIP joint had been previously shown in other joints, including the knee and other hand joints [13, 14].

Based on normal nail histology and MRI in early disease, we have proposed that the pattern of DIP joint-nail disease is better explained as an aberrant inflammatory reaction at sites of mechanical stress, with the epicentre at the enthesis [15]. Attachment points or entheses are sites of high mechanical stress, which is dissipated over a wide area, including the adjacent bone trabecular networks and periosteum of the distal phalanx [16]. We have also noted that large-joint, normal cadaveric entheses demonstrate conspicuous microdamage, microinflammatory changes and associated tissue repair responses, both in the enthesis-bone interface and in the soft tissue components of the enthesis [17, 18].

The combined imaging and anatomical studies indicate that the enthesis is the likely primary basis for joint and skeletal disease localisation in PsA and that other musculoskeletal features, including synovitis and osteitis, can also be conceptualised in relationship to enthesitis [19]. The histological findings of microdamage at normal entheses are reminiscent of the Koebner responses that are well known to dermatologists in the setting of both skin psoriasis and nail disease [20, 21]. The recognition of the functional integration between the nail and enthesis including the bone therefore offers a better understanding of rare psoriatic disease variants, such as acral pustular psoriasis, that have been reported with resorptive osteolysis (deep Koebner phenomenon) [22].

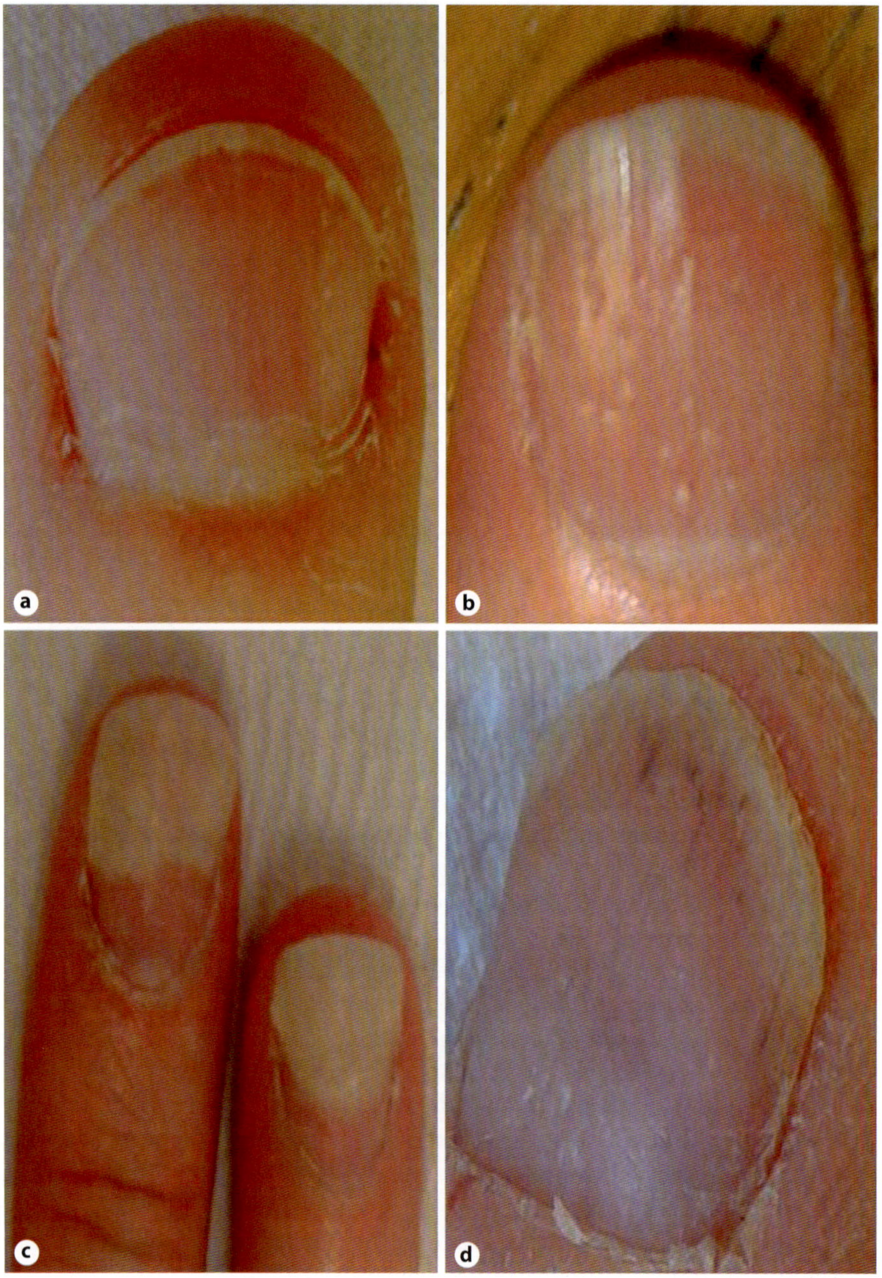

**Fig. 3.** Abnormalities associated with the nail: regular pitting of the nail (**a**), irregular pitting of the nail (**b**), onycholysis (**c**) and splinter haemorrhages (**d**). The common nail matrix changes of pitting and nail bed changes of onycholysis have not been conceptualised in relation to the regional nail-enthesis connections. The extensor tendon is attached to the nail matrix in an interdigitating fashion, which could be relevant to understanding linear pitting. Likewise, the collateral ligaments fuse with a lateral lamina to anchor the nail. It remains to be seen what role these play in nail-related pathology. It seems that some changes, including subungual hyperkeratosis, are related to keratinocyte abnormalities and are not obviously linked to the enthesis.

### Nail Psoriasis Phenotypes: Nail Matrix Lesions

Thus far, the relationship between nail lesions in psoriasis and the nail-enthesis functional unit has not been considered, and these lesions are briefly considered from the enthesis perspective. Dermatologists have long recognised that the clinical features of nail psoriasis can be split into those involving the nail matrix and the nail plate. In the nail matrix, these features include nail pitting, crumbling, splitting and leuconychia. Nail pitting (fig. 3a, b) is indicative of superficial nail abnormalities, and its presence implies that the proximal part of the nail matrix is involved, since this area is responsible for producing the superficial layers of the nail plate. Histologically, the pits often represent local areas of parakeratosis where poorly adherent cells are desquamated from the nail plate [5]. Pits may be randomly distributed or uniformly arranged in series along one or several longitudinal lines or may appear in an orderly crisscross pattern (rippled pitting). Given that the extensor tendon may be attached to the nail matrix in an interdigitating pattern, this could be relevant to understanding linear pitting. Nail plate crumbling suggests extensive involvement of the nail matrix in the psoriatic process [23]. Nail splitting suggests that the distal part of the matrix is implicated, for it is here that the deeper layers of the nail plate are made [5]. Leuconychia may also involve the nail matrix, with the area of involvement thought to be on the undersurface of the nail plate [4]. Electron microscopy studies have shown clear vacuoles located on the white part of the nail; however, they were not seen on the distal part. These observations confirm the probable participation of parakeratosis and keratin abnormalities in this pathology but also suggest an important role of lipid vacuoles [24].

### Nail Psoriasis Phenotypes: Nail Bed Lesions

Onycholysis (separation of the nail plate from the nail bed) (fig. 3c) represents a common nail lesion that is thought to involve the hyponychium. It allows air to get under the distal end of the nail plate, accounting for the whitish colour. Accumulation of large amounts of serum-like exudate containing glycoprotein under the affected nail may explain the colour change in onycholysis [7] and may therefore be linked to keratinocyte dysfunction. The entire nail plate loses its normal mechanical properties and lifts off the nail bed, leaving the latter exposed [25, 26].

'Oily spot' or 'salmon patch' nail plate lesions may start in the middle of the nail. There is usually a yellowish-brown margin visible between the pink, normal nail and the white, oily spot-salmon patch lesion. Nail separation may start here rather than at the hyponychium [4].

Macroscopically, splinter haemorrhages appear as small linear structures, usually not greater than 2 or 3 mm long, arranged at the end of the nail. They are commonly found in the first three fingers of both hands and develop at the line of separation of the nail plate from the nail bed. It is thought that the elongated form of splinter haemorrhages reflects the rupture of wide-calibre vessels beneath the hyponychium and tracking of extravasated blood down the longitudinal furrows beneath the nail plate [5].

We have proposed that the enthesis-nail complex could be a key to understanding different patterns of psoriatic nail disease [11]. However, these nail phenotypes have yet to be explored in relation to perturbation of the enthesis network around the nail, including extensor tendons, the lateral lamina or dermal ligaments. It seems likely that some abnormalities, such as nail hypertrophy and subungual hyperkeratosis, can be fairly clearly linked to the skin phenotype. Whilst this seems to be clearly skin-related, with keratinocyte hyperplasia, it is fair to say that the microanatomical and immunopathological basis for these nail changes in relation to the extensive enthesis network around the fingers is incompletely understood. Certainly, the relationship between nail changes and unrecognised enthesitis in the digits remains to be defined [4, 23, 26, 27]. This is something that high-resolution imaging in man may achieve.

### The Role of Inflammation in Skin and Nail Psoriasis

It is evident that the entire psoriatic disease spectrum has a prominent inflammatory component, but this is difficult to directly investigate in the nail. It is clear from imaging the DIP joints with high-resolution MRI that the nail matrix is involved in the inflammatory response as determined by Gd-DTPA (gadolinium-diethylenetriamine pentaacetic acid) enhancement [11]. However, we are not aware of specific histological studies of the nail matrix in psoriasis subjects with nail disease.

### Imaging to Establish Subclinical Evidence of Enthesitis in Psoriasis

Subclinical enthesitis appears to be very common in patients with psoriasis but not arthritis. Based on more than three decades of research, it has become evident that subjects with psoriasis but without arthritis may have subclinical skeletal-related pathology. The original studies by Namey and Rosenthall [28] showed that subjects with psoriasis had increased isotope uptake along the periosteum – an observation that in hindsight supports the presence of enthesitis and osteitis [29]. Several other studies have replicated this finding, with the most recent ultrasound imaging study showing that subclinical enthesitis of the large joints in the lower limbs was common in subjects with psoriasis, none of whom had joint symptoms [29]. The key question is whether nail disease represents a type of subclinical enthesitis that might be relevant to the future prediction of widespread musculoskeletal disease.

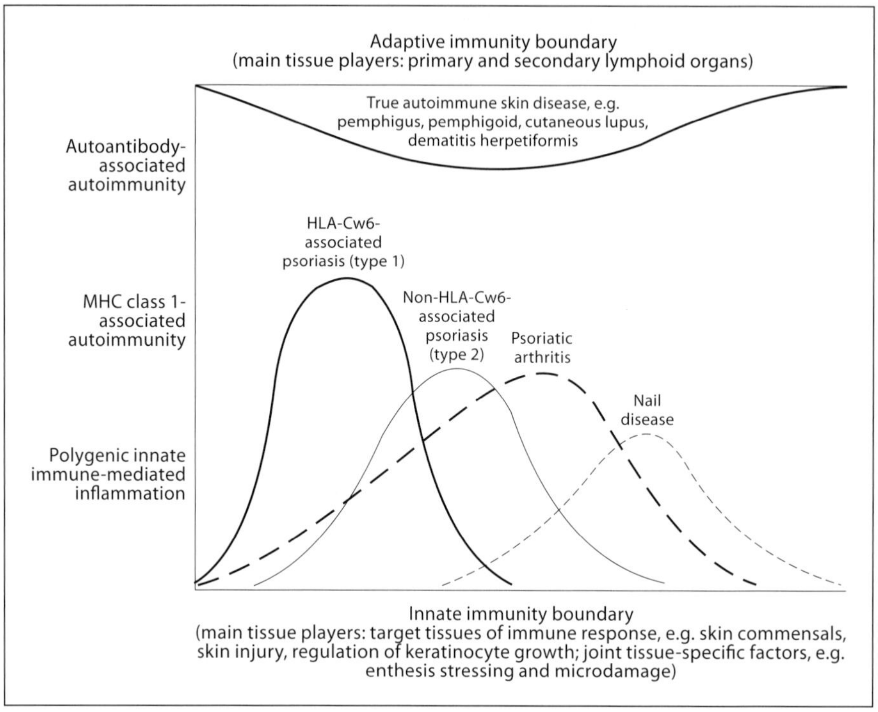


**Fig. 4.** Psoriatic disease spectrum immunological classification. This model is based on the concept of viewing inflammation against self as sitting somewhere along an immunological disease continuum. This figure shows how nail and joint disease appear to be more strongly linked from an immunogenetic perspective than skin and nail disease. Type 1 psoriasis is linked to human leucocyte antigen (HLA)-Cw6, suggesting a major role for adaptive immunity. However, this is radically different from the 'classical' autoantibody-associated autoimmune diseases, in which major histocompatibility complex class II associations and autoantibodies are evident (upper panel). The underlying target tissue molecular abnormalities that lead to persistent innate immune activation at the nail and joint-related entheses have not yet been defined, but aberrant responses to mechanical stressing could be important. It therefore appears that there is a differential involvement of innate and adaptive immunity in the psoriatic disease spectrum.

Indeed, preliminary imaging studies in psoriasis-related pathology have shown a clear link with enthesitis and related osteitis. Psoriatic onychopachydermoperiostitis (POPP) is an uncommon variant of the psoriatic disease spectrum that may present to either rheumatologists or dermatologists. The changes associated with POPP consist of nail dystrophy, periungual swelling and a periosteal reaction in the terminal phalanx on radiography [30–32]. The mechanism of bony damage has been conceptualised in relation to inflammation passing from the subungual dermis to the bone [33, 34]. The MRI description of POPP clearly attests to a nail-enthesis-bone apparatus diffuse inflammatory disorder [35]. This is highly reminiscent of the diffuse digital inflammation, including enthesis-bone involvement, that we have commonly seen in PsA of the DIP joints in the hand [13, 36].

## Common Genetic Traits between Nail and Skin Disease

Thus far, we have argued that there is a common microanatomical basis for joint and nail disease in subjects with psoriatic disease. If this is a tenable theory, then emerging immunogenetics might similarly show a relationship between joint and nail disease but not skin disease. The association of type 1 psoriasis with human leucocyte antigen (HLA)-Cw6 within the major histocompatibility complex appears very robust [37]. Patients with type 1 psoriasis who carry the HLA class I allele HLA-Cw6 not only have an earlier onset, but also more extensive and severe skin disease.

However, it is now evident that nail disease does not share this HLA-Cw6 association, which has been demonstrated in both Caucasian and Chinese populations [38, 39]. Likewise, in a recent case-controlled association study, the HLA-Cw6 phenotype frequencies were compared between patients with PsA and type 1 and 2 psoriasis alone, and it was concluded that carrying the HLA-Cw6 gene was associated with psoriasis alone and not PsA [40]. The same group investigated the interleukin (IL)-23R and IL-12B genetic polymorphisms that have been linked to psoriasis [41]. The group concluded that the recently described IL-23R/IL-12B genetic associations were 'primarily associated with psoriasis susceptibility' [41]. It will be intriguing to see whether psoriasis-related nail disease is linked to the IL-12/IL-23 genetic polymorphisms.

## Improved Classification of Psoriatic Disease Based on an Understanding of the Nail

The classically recognised autoimmune diseases, such as rheumatoid arthritis and diabetes, invariably attack one antigenic territory and progress inexorably until it is destroyed. However, we feel that the pattern of psoriasis and PsA and nail disease points to a radically different immunopathology. Psoriasis has been considered an autoimmune disease. However, there has been a 'swinging pendulum' of academic dermatology research that has oscillated between the concept of a T-cell-mediated disorder versus a keratinocyte-mediated disorder. Based in part on our research in PsA, we have proposed a new classification for human inflammatory disease that is termed the immunological disease continuum [42]. This continuum sets boundaries for adaptive immune-driven disease at one extreme and innate immune-driven disease at the other. This classification scheme accommodates both T-cell and keratinocyte paradigms of psoriasis [43]. Tissue-specific factors, many of which are likely to be ill-defined but include trauma responses and host-microbe interactions, are likely to underscore the psoriatic disease spectrum of disorders. It has further been proposed that in the case of type 1 psoriasis, the innate immune activation taking place in the skin may break tolerance for a specific hitherto undefined antigen, leading to T-cell immunoreactivity [43], and this represents the autoimmune part of the psoriatic disease spectrum. But in the case of nail and joint disease, the innate immune response may play a much greater role in disease [43] (fig. 4).

So far, it appears that T-cell responses are more dominant in skin disease but that innate immune responses are more dominant in joint and nail disease, which is supported by the observation that T-cell-directed therapies may be useful for the skin but not the joints [42]. In support of these concepts, innate immune cytokine pathway blockade with infliximab and other anti-tumour necrosis factor (TNF) agents may be more efficacious in joint and nail disease [44], since lower dosing is more effective than in skin disease, in which a larger dose is generally needed.

## Conclusions

In this article, we argue that a relatively ignored skin and musculoskeletal appendage, the nail, appears to hold the key to understanding the genetic and immunological basis for psoriatic disease. Although much has been written about animal models of psoriasis, these have tended to ignore the nail phenotype in human psoriasis. The advent of high-resolution imaging in man to explore the nail, coupled with emerging immunogenetics and therapies, holds the key to a better understanding of nail disease and indeed systemic disorders that afflict the nail in man. The emerging data showing excellent response of psoriatic nail disease to anti-TNF therapies [44–46] that act principally on the innate arm of the immune response further support the idea of local innate immune responses in the nail-enthesis-bone apparatus as underscoring disease mechanisms at that site.

## Conflicts of Interest

Dennis McGonagle serves as a scientific speaker for Schering Corporation, a subsidiary of Merck & Co., Inc. Editorial support for the development of this publication was provided by Schering Corporation, a subsidiary of Merck & Co., Inc.

## References

1 Wright V: Psoriasis and arthritis. Ann Rheum Dis 1956;15:348–356.
2 Gisondi P, Tinazzi I, El-Dalati G, et al: Lower limb enthesopathy in patients with psoriasis without clinical signs of arthropathy: a hospital-based case-control study. Ann Rheum Dis 2008;67:26–30.
3 Scarpa R, Ayala F, Caporaso N, Olivieri I: Psoriasis, psoriatic arthritis, or psoriatic disease? J Rheumatol 2006;33:210–212.
4 Jiaravuthisan MM, Sasseville D, Vender RB, Murphy F, Muhn CY: Psoriasis of the nail: anatomy, pathology, clinical presentation, and a review of the literature on therapy. J Am Acad Dermatol 2007;57:1–27.
5 Zaias N: Nail in Health and Disease, ed 2. London, Appleton and Lange, 1990.
6 de Berker DA, Andre J, Baran R: Nail biology and nail science. Int J Cosmet Sci 2007;29: 241–275.

7 Fleckman P: Structure and function of the nail unit; in Scher RK, Daniel CR III (eds): Nails: Diagnosis, Therapy, Surgery, ed 3. Philadelphia, Elsevier, 2005, pp 13–26.
8 Martin BF, Platts MM: A histological study of the nail region in normal human subjects and in those showing splinter haemorrhages of the nail. J Anat 1959;93:323–330.
9 Frenz C, Fritsch H, Hoch J: Plastination histologic investigations on the inserting pars terminalis aponeurosis dorsalis of three-sectioned fingers. Ann Anat 2000;182:69–73.
10 Tan AL, Benjamin M, Toumi H, et al: The relationship between the extensor tendon enthesis and the nail in distal interphalangeal joint disease in psoriatic arthritis – a high-resolution MRI and histological study. Rheumatology (Oxford) 2007;46:253–256.
11 McGonagle D, Tan AL, Benjamin M: The nail as a musculoskeletal appendage – implications for an improved understanding of the link between psoriasis and arthritis. Dermatology 2009;218:97–102.
12 Tan AL, Grainger AJ, Tanner SF, Emery P, McGonagle D: A high-resolution magnetic resonance imaging study of distal interphalangeal joint arthropathy in psoriatic arthritis and osteoarthritis: are they the same? Arthritis Rheum 2006;54:1328–1333.
13 McGonagle D, Gibbon W, O'Connor P, Green M, Pease C, Emery P: Characteristic magnetic resonance imaging entheseal changes of knee synovitis in spondylarthropathy. Arthritis Rheum 1998;41:694–700.
14 Jevtic V, Watt I, Rozman B, Kos-Golja M, Demsar F, Jarh O: Distinctive radiological features of small hand joints in rheumatoid arthritis and seronegative spondyloarthritis demonstrated by contrast-enhanced (Gd-DTPA) magnetic resonance imaging. Skeletal Radiol 1995;24:351–355.
15 McGonagle D: Imaging the joint and enthesis: insights into pathogenesis of psoriatic arthritis. Ann Rheum Dis 2005;64:ii58–ii60.
16 Benjamin M, McGonagle D: The anatomical basis for disease localisation in seronegative spondyloarthropathy at entheses and related sites. J Anat 2001;199:503–526.
17 Benjamin M, McGonagle D: Histopathologic changes at 'synovio-entheseal complexes' suggesting a novel mechanism for synovitis in osteoarthritis and spondylarthritis. Arthritis Rheum 2007;56:3601–3609.
18 Benjamin M, Toumi H, Suzuki D, Redman S, Emery P, McGonagle D: Microdamage and altered vascularity at the enthesis-bone interface provides an anatomic explanation for bone involvement in the HLA-B27-associated spondylarthritides and allied disorders. Arthritis Rheum 2007;56:224–233.
19 McGonagle D, Lories RJ, Tan AL, Benjamin M: The concept of a 'synovio-entheseal complex' and its implications for understanding joint inflammation and damage in psoriatic arthritis and beyond. Arthritis Rheum 2007;56:2482–2491.
20 Raychaudhuri SP, Jiang WY, Raychaudhuri SK: Revisiting the Koebner phenomenon: role of NGF and its receptor system in the pathogenesis of psoriasis (comment). Am J Pathol 2008;172:961–971.
21 Baker BS, Powles AV, Lambert S, Valdimarsson H, Fry L: A prospective study of the Koebner reaction and T lymphocytes in uninvolved psoriatic skin. Acta Derm Venereol 1988;68:430–434.
22 Sahin GO, Akyol M, Ozcelik S: An unusual Koebner phenomenon secondary to PPD with pustular and arthropathic psoriasis. Eur J Dermatol 2007;17:446.
23 Fawcett RS, Linford S, Stulberg DL: Nail abnormalities: clues to systemic disease. Am Fam Physician 2004;69:1417–1424.
24 Marcilly MC, Balme B, Haftek M, et al: Subtotal hereditary leukonychia, histopathological and electron microscopy study of 'milky' nails. Ann Dermatol Venereol 2003;130:50–54.
25 Samman PD, Fenton DA (eds): The Nail in Disease. London, William Heinemann, 1986.
26 Baran R, Dawber RPR (eds): Diseases of the Nail and Their Management. Oxford, Blackwell Scientific Publications, 1984.
27 Lewin K, DeWit S, Ferrington RA: Pathology of the finger nail in psoriasis: a clinicopathological study. Br J Dermatol 1972;86:555–563.
28 Namey TC, Rosenthall L: Periarticular uptake of 99mtechnetium diphosphonate in psoriatics: correlation with cutaneous activity. Arthritis Rheum 1976;19:607–612.
29 McGonagle D, Marzo-Ortega H, Benjamin M, Emery P: Report on the Second International Enthesitis Workshop. Arthritis Rheum 2003;48:896–905.
30 Mahoney JM, Scott R: Psoriatic onychopachydermoperiostitis (POPP): a perplexing case study. J Am Podiatr Med Assoc 2009;99:140–143.
31 Resnick D, Broderick TW: Bony proliferation of terminal toe phalanges in psoriasis: the 'ivory' phalanx. J Can Assoc Radiol 1977;28:187–189.
32 McGonagle D, Conaghan PG, Emery P: Psoriatic arthritis: a unified concept twenty years on. Arthritis Rheum 1999;42:1080–1086.
33 Jury CS, Fleming C, Kemmett D: Severe nail dystrophy associated with painful fingertips. Diagnosis: psoriatic onychopachydermoperiostitis (POPP). Arch Dermatol 2000;136:925–930.
34 Srivastava M, Solomon G, Strober B: Psoriatic onycho-pachydermo periostitis. Dermatol Online J 2007;13:20.
35 Bongartz T, Harle P, Friedrich S, et al: Successful treatment of psoriatic onycho-pachydermo periostitis (POPP) with adalimumab. Arthritis Rheum 2005;52:280–282.
36 Marzo-Ortega H, McGonagle D, Rhodes LA, et al: Efficacy of infliximab on MRI-determined bone oedema in psoriatic arthritis. Ann Rheum Dis 2007;66:778–781.
37 Elder JT: Genome-wide association scan yields new insights into the immunopathogenesis of psoriasis. Genes Immun 2009;10:201–209.
38 Gudjonsson JE, Karason A, Antonsdottir AA, et al: HLA-Cw6-positive and HLA-Cw6-negative patients with psoriasis vulgaris have distinct clinical features. J Invest Dermatol 2002;118:362–365.
39 Fan X, Yang S, Sun LD, et al: Comparison of clinical features of HLA-Cw*0602-positive and -negative psoriasis patients in a Han Chinese population. Acta Derm Venereol 2007;87:335–340.
40 Ho PY, Barton A, Worthington J, Thomson W, Silman AJ, Bruce IN: HLA-Cw6 and HLA-DRB1*07 together are associated with less severe joint disease in psoriatic arthritis. Ann Rheum Dis 2007;66:807–811.
41 Filer C, Ho P, Smith RL, et al: Investigation of association of the IL12B and IL23R genes with psoriatic arthritis. Arthritis Rheum 2008;58:3705–3709.
42 McGonagle D, McDermott MF: A proposed classification of the immunological diseases. PLoS Med 2006;3:e297.
43 McGonagle D, Georgouli T: The importance of 'Mechnikov's thorn' for an improved understanding of 21st century medicine and immunology: a view from the eye. Scand J Immunol 2008;68:129–139.
44 Lawry M: Biological therapy and nail psoriasis. Dermatol Ther 2007;20:60–67.
45 Rigopoulos D, Gregoriou S, Stratigos A, et al: Evaluation of the efficacy and safety of infliximab on psoriatic nails: an unblinded, nonrandomized, open-label study. Br J Dermatol 2008;159:453–456.
46 Rich P, Griffiths CEM, Reich K, et al: Baseline nail disease in patients with moderate to severe psoriasis and response to treatment with infliximab during 1 year. J Am Acad Dermatol 2008;58:224–231.

Dermatology

Dermatology 2010;221(suppl 1):23–28
DOI: 10.1159/000316177

Published online: August 9, 2010

# Methods of Outcomes Measurement in Nail Psoriasis

M. Augustin[a] A. Ogilvie[b]

[a]Center for Health Services Research in Dermatology (CVderm), Department of Dermatology, University Clinics of Hamburg, Hamburg, and [b]Psoriasis Clinic, Department of Dermatology, University Clinics of Erlangen, Erlangen, Germany

**Key Words**

Nail psoriasis · Assessment tools · Psoriasis

**Abstract**

***Background:*** Nail involvement is a common feature of psoriasis, predicting higher disease severity and greater impairment in quality of life. Valid assessment of nail psoriasis is relevant for research and routine clinical use. However, no measurement standards have currently been developed. ***Objective:*** To identify state-of-the-art outcomes measurements in nail psoriasis by literature analysis. ***Methods:*** Systematic Web-based literature search, followed by structured critical appraisal and consecutive descriptive report. The search focused on methodological and epidemiological publications and papers describing outcomes of clinical trials on nail psoriasis. ***Results:*** Initially, 646 publications met the primary criteria. After non-relevant or replicate publications were excluded, 66 papers were analysed, including clinical trials or case reports (n = 41), reviews (n = 11) and methodological or epidemiological studies (n = 14). In total, 23 clinical outcomes measures and 15 patient-reported outcomes (PRO) tools were used. None had been validated according to recent standards. In the studies with clinical interventions (n = 41), NAPSI (Nail Psoriasis Severity Index; n = 4) or target NAPSI (n = 2) were the most often used single tools, followed by Physician's Global Assessment (n = 3). However, in 16 studies, no specifically described outcomes measures were used. ***Conclusion:*** Valid clinical outcomes measures in nail psoriasis are rare. Existing tools lack validation and standardisation. A need exists for accurate and scientifically sound evaluation of nail psoriasis severity in trials and clinical practice. To cover all elements of nail psoriasis, the optimal nail psoriasis assessment tool would include both PRO and physician-assessed outcomes measures.



## Introduction

With a prevalence of 2–3%, psoriasis vulgaris is one of the most common chronic skin diseases [1, 2]. Due to the serious impairments in quality of life caused by the usually chronic and often refractory course of disease, psoriasis is of considerable socioeconomic relevance [3, 4]. Additionally, different types of diseases are associated with psoriasis. For example, there is a distinct pattern of enthesitis, osteitis and synovitis that is generally referred to as psoriatic arthritis (PsA) [5–7]. Recent data from two distinct trials suggest that approximately 20% of German patients visiting a dermatologist for psoriasis have PsA [8, 9]. Moreover, in approximately 85% of these cases, PsA

KARGER

Fax +41 61 306 12 34
E-Mail karger@karger.ch
www.karger.com


1018–8665/10/2215–0023$26.00/0

Accessible online at:
www.karger.com/drm

Prof. Dr. med. Matthias Augustin, MD
Center for Health Services Research in Dermatology (CVderm)
Department of Dermatology, University Clinics of Hamburg
Martinistrasse 52, DE–20246 Hamburg (Germany)
Tel. +49 40 42803 5428, Fax +49 40 42803 5348, E-Mail m.augustin@derma.de

was newly diagnosed, even with previous complaints of joint problems [8]. Several studies have also demonstrated that patients with psoriasis can have an increased risk of developing comorbidities related to the metabolic syndrome [2, 10]. The most frequent association of psoriasis and concomitant disease, however, is found with nail psoriasis. Variable prevalence data demonstrate that up to 50% of patients with psoriasis have concurrent nail psoriasis [11–13]. In patients with moderate to severe psoriasis, approximately 82% have symptoms of nail psoriasis [14]; up to 5% of patients have nail psoriasis alone [11–12]. In most cases, a diagnosis of nail psoriasis is established according to clinical criteria; thus, it is important to examine the complete integument to understand its burden on the patient.

Evaluating the severity of nail involvement in psoriasis remains challenging. A variety of systems have been established to evaluate nail psoriasis, including Baran's nail psoriasis severity index [15], Cannavò's scoring system [16] and the nail psoriasis quality of life scale (NPQ10) [17]. The Nail Psoriasis Severity Index (NAPSI) is a reproducible, objective and simple tool for the clinical assessment of psoriatic nail disease and is the only clinical scale that has been validated [18]. As with other tools, the NAPSI has limitations in terms of sensitivity and exclusion of types of changes and degree of severity [18, 19]. Moreover, nail psoriasis can cause both physical and psychological impairments that significantly reduce health-related quality of life (HRQoL) [13]. For these reasons, any assessment of nail psoriasis severity should include HRQoL parameters from the patient's perspective. To date, none of the existing assessment tools for nail psoriasis address both objective and patient-reported parameters.

Only recently, publications have focused on the question of validity and feasibility in outcomes measurements of nail psoriasis [20–23]. The objective of this study was to identify state-of-the-art outcomes measurements of nail psoriasis by a literature search.

## Methods

*Study Design*

The study was designed as a literature review of publications based on a protocol-driven search of online databases with a concurrent consecutive manual search. The literature search was completed by July 2009. Data analysis was descriptive and was performed by CVderm. All databases were searched from their inception to the date of the search. Searches were also undertaken of several Internet-accessible data sources (fig. 1). The bibliographies of all publications were reviewed to identify further relevant studies. Hand-searching continued throughout the project. The terms for the search strategies were identified through discussion between two Cochrane specialists from CVderm and the authors (M.A., A.O.) by scanning the background literature and several health technology assessment reports on psoriasis and by browsing the MEDLINE thesaurus (MeSH). The systematic search of PubMed was performed as described in figure 2.

- MEDLINE and In-Process Citations (PubMed Online) (http://www.ashburypress.com/medline/resources/in-process.html)
- EMBASE (Ovid Online) (http://www.ovid.com/site/products/ovidguide/embase.htm)
- Cochrane Central Register of Controlled Trials (CENTRAL) (http://uscc.cochrane.org/en/index.html)
- CenterWatch (http://www.centerwatch.com/)
- Current Controlled Trials (http://controlled-trials.com/)
- ClinicalTrials.gov (http://clinicaltrials.gov/)
- NHS Economic Evaluation Database (NHS EED) (CRD administration database) (http://www.crd.york.ac.uk/crdweb/Home.aspx?DB=NHS%20EED)
- EconLit (SilverPlatter on the Web) (http://www.accessmylibrary.com/web-econlit-silverplatter.html)
- ISI Science and Technology Proceedings (http://wos.mimas.ac.uk/)
- Social Sciences Citation Index (http://wos.mimas.ac.uk/)
- Science Citation Index (http://wos.mimas.ac.uk/)

**Fig. 1.** Internet search databases used in the literature search.

*Study Selection*

Two reviewers (M.A., A.O.) independently selected the studies for review based on the paper titles and abstracts. Discrepancies were resolved by consensus, and a third reviewer was consulted if necessary. Studies reported as full publications or unpublished full reports were included in the review. Studies reported as abstracts were included only if adequate information was provided. All titles and abstracts identified by the search were screened, and any references that were considered relevant by either reviewer were obtained. No language or other restrictions were applied. Only publications that included specific information on the use of instruments for the diagnosis or assessment of nail psoriasis were considered.

*Critical Appraisal*

The included publications were analysed according to a structured protocol and transferred into a predesigned Excel form. The criteria for analysis referred to the following questions:

- Are there any publications on the methodology of outcomes measurement in nail psoriasis, and if yes, are there any validation data on these methods?
- Which outcomes parameters are used in clinical trials on nail psoriasis?
- Which parameters were used in studies on epidemiology of nail psoriasis?

*Data Extraction Strategy*

All data were extracted by one reviewer and independently checked for accuracy by the second reviewer. Disagreements were resolved through consensus and by consultation with a third reviewer if necessary. Data from studies with multiple publications were extracted and reported as from a single study. The following details were extracted from each trial (if applicable):

- Study details (author, year, country, type of publication, other publications/reports, study design, setting, duration of trial follow-up, frequency of follow-up, sample size calculation, analyses).
- Participant details (number randomised and treated, age, gender, psoriasis history, duration of psoriasis and nail psoriasis, proportion of patients with nail affection).
- Clinical characterisation of patients, e.g. Psoriasis Area and Severity Index, Dermatology Life Quality Index (DLQI), body surface area at baseline.
- Details of outcomes measurements.

*Assessment of Study Quality*

The quality of trials was assessed by one reviewer and independently checked by a second reviewer. Disagreements were resolved through consensus, and a third reviewer was consulted if necessary.

*Efficacy Trials*

The efficacy trials were assessed for quality using a checklist compiled from criteria specified in the methodology of the German Federal Joint Committee (Gemeinsamer Bundesausschuss). The quality of each study was summarised as a quality rating, classifying trials as excellent, good, satisfactory or poor.

*Epidemiological Studies and Economic Evaluations*

Data were extracted into a quality assessment template, covering selection of alternatives, treatment of costs and benefits (including any modelling undertaken), use of discounting, allowance for uncertainty and presentation of results. The checklist is an updated version of that developed by Drummond et al. [24].

## Results

*Systematic Literature Search*

Based on the strategy outlined above, 104 publications were found that included the combination of nail psoriasis and outcomes measurement (fig. 3). Thirty-eight publications had to be excluded for the following reasons: irrelevant for research questions, replicate publications and no outcomes measured. Sixty-six publications were selected for analysis (table 1). These included 41 clinical publications and 25 publications without clinical data collection. The latter consisted of 11 reviews and 14 methodological or epidemiological studies. The clinical publications included 27 clinical trials and 14 other publications addressing clinical outcomes.

Group 1
1. Nail psoriasis

Group 2
2. Outcome
3. Endpoint
4. Severity
5. Measure
6. Method
7. Quality of life
8. Patient-reported outcomes
9. Patient benefit
10. Disease burden
11. Psychology
12. Distress
13. Score

Pool: (#2 OR #3 … OR #13)

Papers to be analysed: #1 AND (#2 OR #3 … OR #13)

Group 3 for the further characterisation of papers identified
14. Clinical trial
15. Randomised clinical trial
16. Epidemiology
17. Review

**Fig. 2.** Systematic search of PubMed.

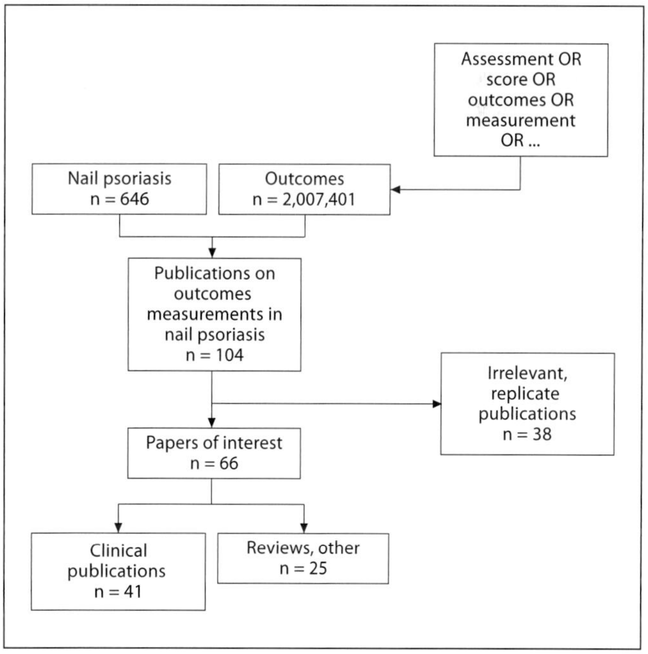


**Fig. 3.** Results of the literature search on nail psoriasis and outcomes measures.

**Table 1.** Publications regarding the epidemiology of nail psoriasis or the methodology of nail psoriasis outcomes measurement

| | |
|---|---|
| Clinical trials | |
| Uncontrolled clinical trials | 9 |
| Randomised controlled trials | 10 |
| Non-randomised controlled trials | 8 |
| Total | 27 |
| Treatment evaluations | |
| Retrospective data analyses | 5 |
| Non-interventional studies | 7 |
| Safety trials | 0 |
| Case studies | 2 |
| Total | 14 |
| Nonclinical publications | |
| Literature review | 7 |
| Systematic review | 4 |
| Methodological study | 2 |
| Epidemiological survey | 1 |
| Other | 11 |
| Total | 25 |
| Total publications | |
| Clinical trials | 27 |
| Treatment evaluations | 14 |
| Non-clinical publications | 25 |
| Total | 66 |

**Table 2.** Characteristics of nail psoriasis in the clinical publications (n = 41)

| | Clinical trials | Treatment evaluations | All clinical publications |
|---|---|---|---|
| Publications | 27 | 14 | 41 |
| Patients | 2,824 | 6,564 | 9,388 |
| Nail Pso patients, % | 87.4 | 69.4 | 76.5 |
| History of psoriasis, years | 14.9 | 14.1 | 14.4 |
| History of Nail Pso, years | 10.0 | NA | 10.0 |
| PsA patients, total, % | 54.0 | 43.3 | 44.5 |
| PsA among Nail Pso, % | 4.0 | 73.6 | 68.2 |
| Mean age, Nail Pso, years | 50.9 | 37.3 | 42.7 |
| Mean age, no Nail Pso, years | 48.6 | 33.3 | 32.9 |
| Male patients, Nail Pso, % | 77.4 | 51.7 | 65.7 |
| Male patients, no Nail Pso, % | 11.5 | 76.6 | 49.4 |

PsA = Psoriatic arthritis; Nail Pso = nail psoriasis.

*Outcomes Tools in Epidemiological and Methodological Studies*

In the literature search, 3% (2/66) of the publications selected covered the methodology of nail psoriasis evaluation. These publications included the development of instruments for nail assessment. However, these assessments were not based on international standards of test development but were performed on a clinical basis.

*Outcomes Tools in Clinical Trials*

In the clinical trials, a total of 9,388 patients were observed (table 2). Since the clinical characteristics in the trials are subject to selection bias, no epidemiological conclusions from the data can be drawn. Regarding the clinical publications, there were two instruments mentioned that specifically evaluated the clinical severity of nail psoriasis: the NAPSI (n = 4) or target NAPSI (n = 2), and Cannavò's score (n = 1). In the review another severity score was named, nail area severity score, but not indicated as used. However, in most clinical studies and in the case reports, no specific instruments for the assessment of patient-reported outcomes (PRO) were found (n = 14). PRO were measured in 24% (10/41) of the studies. In these cases, disease-specific, but not condition-specific, quality of life instruments were used. Surprisingly, data on DLQI were not reported in any of the publications.

In total, 14 clinical trials were identified that assessed nail psoriasis under treatment (table 3). Nine of these trials focused directly on nail psoriasis; the others looked at psoriasis in general (n = 4) or at several indications (n = 1).

## Discussion

The present investigation was performed to obtain an overview of outcomes instruments used in nail psoriasis. Clinical outcomes studies as well as methodological or epidemiological studies were included. A total of 66 publications met the inclusion criteria, indicating that outcomes assessments in nail psoriasis have not yet been frequently performed. The number of clinical trials with a specific focus on nail psoriasis is low. Moreover, only a few publications addressed the question of valid measurement for nail psoriasis, though some have explored the correlation between instruments. For example, EXPRESS (European Infliximab for Psoriasis [Remicade®] Efficacy and Safety Study) demonstrated that the number of nails involved and target nail NAPSI scores correlated significantly at baseline and during treatment

**Table 3.** Outcomes measures used in the clinical studies (n = 41 publications)

| | Clinical trials | Treatment evaluations | All clinical publications |
|---|---|---|---|
| Publications | 27 | 14 | 41 |
| Total patients | 2,824 | 6,564 | 9,388 |
| Patients per study, mean | 157 | 298 | 232 |
| Clinical scores on nail psoriasis | 15 | 11 | 26 |
| Total NAPSI | 3 | 1 | 4 |
| Target NAPSI | 0 | 2 | 2 |
| Cannavò | 1 | 0 | 1 |
| NAS | 0 | 0 | 0 |
| Other score | 7 | 7 | 14 |
| Nail count | 1 | 1 | 2 |
| PGA dyn | 1 | 0 | 1 |
| PGA stat | 2 | 0 | 2 |
| Patient-reported outcomes | 7 | 3 | 10 |
| PatGA dyn | 2 | 0 | 2 |
| PatGA stat | 3 | 1 | 4 |
| Burden of disease | 1 | 0 | 1 |
| QoL – DLQI | 0 | 0 | 0 |
| QoL – other | 1 | 2 | 3 |

DLQI = Dermatology Life Quality Index; NAPSI = Nail Psoriasis Severity Index; NAS = nail area severity score; PatGA = Patient's Global Assessment; PGA = Physician's Global Assessment; QoL = quality of life.

with infliximab [25]. Although some correlations may exist, none of the instruments used in any of the trials meet the criteria for outcomes measurement as required, for example, by the German national guidelines [26]. Additionally, no comprehensive PRO measurements specific to nail psoriasis have yet been validated, though a recent publication on nail QoL outcomes measurement demonstrates initial progress [17]. However, the data collected in this review indicate that no specific assessment tools address all disease aspects, including nail severity and the impact of nail psoriasis on HRQoL. As a result, the impact of nail disease in a psoriasis patient may be inadequately measured or underestimated. There is a definite need for more methodological developments in nail psoriasis assessment. A more feasible tool is needed that can serve as an individual measurement of treatment outcomes in clinical trials and also address the importance of adequately evaluating the impact of nail psoriasis on a patient's quality of life in routine practice.

## Conflicts of Interest

M. Augustin and A. Ogilvie serve as consultants for Schering Corporation, a subsidiary of Merck & Co., Inc. Editorial support for the development of this publication was provided by Schering Corporation, a subsidiary of Merck & Co., Inc.

## References

1 Schäfer I, Rustenbach SJ, Zimmer L, Augustin M: Prevalence of skin diseases in a cohort of 48,665 employees in Germany. Dermatology 2008;217:169–172.
2 Augustin M, Reich K, Glaeske G, Schaefer I, Radtke M: Comorbidity and age-related prevalence of psoriasis: analysis of health insurance data in Germany. Acta Derm Venereol 2010;90:147–151.
3 Krueger G, Koo J, Lebwohl M, Menter A, Stern RS, Rolstad T: The impact of psoriasis on quality of life: results of a 1998 National Psoriasis Foundation patient-membership survey. Arch Dermaology 2001;137:280–284.
4 Augustin M, Krüger K, Radtke MA, Schwippl I, Reich K: Disease severity, quality of life and health care in plaque-type psoriasis: a multicenter prospective cross-sectional study in Germany. Dermatology 2008;216:366–372.
5 Henseler T, Christophers E: Disease concomitance in psoriasis. J Am Acad Dermatol 1995;32:982–986.
6 Taylor W, Gladman D, Helliwell P, Marchesoni A, Mease P, Mielants H; CASPAR Study Group: Classification criteria for psoriatic arthritis: development of new criteria from a large international study. Arthritis Rheum 2006;54:2665–2673.
7 Alamanos Y, Voulgari PV, Drosos AA: Incidence and prevalence of psoriatic arthritis: a systematic review. J Rheumatol 2008;35:1354–1358.
8 Reich K, Krüger K, Mössner R, Augustin M: Epidemiology and clinical pattern of psoriatic arthritis in Germany: a prospective interdisciplinary epidemiological study of 1,511 patients with plaque-type psoriasis. Br J Dermatol 2009;160:1040–1047.
9 Radtke MA, Reich K, Blome C, Rustenbach S, Augustin M: Prevalence and clinical features of psoriatic arthritis and joint complaints in 2,009 patients with psoriais: results of a German national survey. J Eur Acad Dermatol Venereol 2009;23:683–691.
10 Sterry W, Strober BE, Menter A; on behalf of the International Psoriasis Council: Obesity in psoriasis: the metabolic, clinical and therapeutic implications. Report of an interdisciplinary conference and review. Br J Dermatol 2007;157:649–655.
11 Farber EM, Nall L: Nail psoriasis. Cutis 1992;50:174–178.
12 Van Laborde S, Scher RK: Developments in the treatment of nail psoriasis, melanonychia striata, and onychomycosis. Dermatol Clin 2000;18:37–46.
13 Augustin M, Reich K, Blome C, Schäfer I, Laass A, Radtke MA: Nail psoriasis in Germany: Epidemiology and burden of disease. Br J Dermatol 2010, Epub ahead of print.
14 Rich P, Griffiths CEM, Reich K, Nestle FO, Scher RK, Li S, Xu S, Hsu MC, Guzzo C: Baseline nail disease in patients with moderate to severe psoriasis and response to treatment with infliximab during 1 year. J Am Acad Dermatol 2008;58:224–231.
15 Baran RL: A nail psoriasis severity index. Br J Dermatol 2004;150:568–569.

16 Cannavò SP, Guarneri F, Vaccaro M, Borgia F, Guarneri B: Treatment of psoriatic nails with topical cyclosporin: a prospective, randomized placebo-controlled study. Dermatology 2003;206:153–156.
17 Ortonne JP, Baran R, Corvest M, Schmitt C, Voisard JJ, Taieb C: Development and validation of nail psoriasis quality of life scale (NPQ10). J Eur Acad Dermatol Venereol 2010;24:22–27.
18 Rich P, Scher RK: Nail Psoriasis Severity Index: a useful tool for evaluation of nail psoriasis. J Am Acad Dermatol 2003;49:206–212.
19 Lawry M: Biological therapy and nail psoriasis. Dermatol Ther 2007;20:60–67.
20 Kacar N, Ergin S, Erdogan BS: The comparison of Nail Psoriasis Severity Index with a less time-consuming qualitative system. J Eur Acad Dermatol Venereol 2008;22:219–222.
21 Cassell SE, Bieber JD, Rich P, Tutuncu ZN, Lee SJ, Kalunian KC, Wu CW, Kavanaugh A: The modified Nail Psoriasis Severity Index: validation of an instrument to assess psoriatic nail involvement in patients with psoriatic arthritis. J Rheumatol 2007;34:123–129.
22 Aktan S, Ilknur T, Akin C, Ozkan S: Interobserver reliability of the Nail Psoriasis Severity Index. Clin Exp Dermatol 2007;32:141–144.
23 Gupta AK, Cooper EA: Psoriatic nail disease: quality of life and treatment. J Cutan Med Surg 2009;13(suppl 2):S102–S106.
24 Drummond MF, O'Brien BJ, Stoddart GL, Torrance GW: Methods for the Economic Evaluation of Health Care Programmes, ed 2. Oxford, Oxford Medical Publications, 1997.
25 Kerkmann U, Winkelman W, Wang Y, Reich K: Target nail NAPSI correlates with number of nails involved: a clinically efficient, useful, and precise assessment for nail psoriasis severity (poster). Presented at the 18th Congress of the European Academy of Dermatology and Venereology, 7–11 October 2009, Berlin, Germany, poster 1164.
26 Augustin M, Amon U, Braathen L, Bullinger M, Gieler U, Klein GF, Schultz-Amling W: Assessment of quality of life in dermatology (German national guideline). J Dtsch Dermatol Ges 2004;9:802–806.

Dermatology

Dermatology 2010;221(suppl 1):29–42
DOI: 10.1159/000316179

Published online: August 9, 2010

# Treatment and Management of Psoriasis with Nail Involvement: A Focus on Biologic Therapy

Richard G. Langley[a] Esteban Daudén[b]

[a]Dalhousie University, Halifax, N.S., Canada; [b]Hospital Universitario de la Princesa, Madrid, Spain

**Key Words**
Biologics · Nail disease · Nail psoriasis · Psoriasis, treatment

**Abstract**
Nail involvement in psoriasis is typically overlooked, although it can affect up to 50% of patients with psoriasis and cause functional impact as well as psychological stress that can significantly affect quality of life. In addition, psoriatic patients with nail disease tend to have a more severe skin condition, a higher rate of unremitting and progressive arthritis and more associated anxiety and depression. Historically, the treatment of nail psoriasis has proven difficult, with most patients feeling that the treatment for their nail disease was unsatisfactory. The current management of nail psoriasis includes topical, intralesional and systemic therapies, although little clinical evidence is available on the effectiveness of conventional treatments and, consequently, no specific treatment approach has been fully supported. Biologic agents are beginning to emerge as a viable option to treat patients with both cutaneous and nail clinical manifestations of psoriasis and psoriatic arthritis. The extra disease burden that nail symptoms place on the patient can be considered indicative of a more severe form of the disease and should be taken into consideration when assessing treatment options. 

## Introduction: Difficulty in Treating Psoriasis with Nail Involvement

Psoriasis is a chronic, incurable skin disease that causes significant distress and morbidity [1, 2]. The severity of psoriasis varies considerably from mild localised distribution to more severe erythrodermic forms [1]. Although the most characteristic findings of psoriasis are skin manifestations, another commonly recognised characteristic is nail involvement. The clinical manifestations associated with nail psoriasis are different in their representations and correlate with the anatomical location of the nail unit that is affected by the disease. If the nail disease stems from the nail matrix, possible representations are leuconychia, red spots, pitting and crumbling. If the nail disease is derived from the nail bed, possible manifestations are oil-drop discolouration, splinter haemorrhages, subungual hyperkeratosis and onycholysis [1]. The most common clinical manifestation is pitting, although others are more severe and can greatly impact the function of the patient.

Nail psoriasis can occur in up to 50% of psoriasis patients, with a lifetime incidence estimated to be between 80 and 90% [3]. Only 5–10% of nail psoriasis cases are thought to occur in the absence of cutaneous disease [4]. Nail disease is more common in patients with more se-

KARGER

Fax +41 61 306 12 34
E-Mail karger@karger.ch
www.karger.com


1018–8665/10/2215–0029$26.00/0

Accessible online at:
www.karger.com/drm

Richard Langley, MD
4195 Dickson Building, Queen Elizabeth II Health Sciences Centre
Dalhousie University, 1278 University Avenue
Halifax, NS B3H 2Y9 (Canada)
Tel. +1 902 425 8038, Fax +1 902 431 8882, E-Mail richard.langley@dal.ca

vere disease – for example, up to 80% of patients with psoriatic arthritis (PsA) often have nail involvement as part of their condition and, as with psoriasis patients, many rarely receive treatment for nail disease [5, 6]. A high association between PsA and nail psoriasis has been noted in several studies [6–14]. In fact, a large population-based cohort study of 1,633 psoriasis patients found that psoriasis subjects with nail dystrophy are almost three times more likely to develop PsA than subjects without nail dystrophy [11].

Nail psoriasis can cause significant physical impairment and pain [6, 7]. Additionally, the compromised nails with psoriasis may also be susceptible to fungal infections [2]. Patients with nail psoriasis typically complain about an altered sense of touch and/or a lack of ability to grab small objects, tie shoelaces and button clothes [4]. In a survey of 7,000 psoriasis sufferers, 1,369 suffered from nail psoriasis. When asked about their nail symptoms, more than 90% of respondents with nail disease found the clinical signs of nail psoriasis cosmetically disturbing [7]. A considerable number also admitted to being restricted in their daily activities, housekeeping and/or profession as a consequence of their nail psoriasis [7]. Importantly, these patients often found the treatments for nail psoriasis disappointing, and 77% said that they would like to use therapy for their nail problems if it were more effective [7].

## Conventional Treatment Approaches to Managing Nail Psoriasis

Nail disease is often overlooked in the management of patients with psoriasis, with cutaneous lesions often being the principal motivation to seek treatment. One difficulty in the treatment of nail psoriasis is that the options are far more limited in scope and efficacy than those for skin manifestations [1]. Nail psoriasis tends to be persistent and refractory to treatment, and many treatment modalities are tedious to administer, with short-lived remissions. The choice of treatment for nail psoriasis depends on the clinical features of the disease and patient-specific features [4]. The clinical evidence for nail psoriasis treatments is sparse, and properly conducted randomised controlled trials are historically rare. The published evidence for various treatment modalities in nail psoriasis is reviewed here. Most trials lack a blinded comparator, raising the possibility of bias and more favourable outcomes than might be observed with a more conservative study design. It is noteworthy that there is a lack of consistency in the outcome measures used, making comparisons of treatment efficacies extremely difficult.

### *Topical Therapies*

Although topical therapy has been a mainstay of treatment for skin psoriasis, its use on nails has been poorly documented [1]. If nail changes are mild and not bothersome to the patient or if nail psoriasis is the sole manifestation of the disease, topical therapies are often an appropriate first choice [4]. The most popular choices of topical therapy for nail psoriasis remain topical glucocorticosteroids and vitamin D3 analogues such as calcipotriol, despite a lack of evidence for efficacy and standardised therapeutic regimens. However, it is common for high-potency topical steroids to be applied to the nails and periungual regions and then covered by occlusive dressings [15, 16]. Other topical agents with limited evidence for efficacy include topical ciclosporin, tazarotene, 5-fluorouracil and anthralin [4].

Response to topical therapy is variable and depends in large part on the anatomical location of psoriasis within the nail unit. For example, if psoriasis affects the nail matrix, treatment is often applied to the nail folds, but if psoriasis is derived from the nail bed, the nails need to be trimmed to the hyponychium before treatment is applied [1]. Also, topical therapies often have adverse effects, including skin atrophy and irritation. Moreover, the use of topical therapies is often unpleasant and inconvenient to patients, and compliance is usually challenging.

The published evidence for topical treatment modalities in nail psoriasis is summarised in table 1.

#### *Calcipotriol and Topical Glucocorticosteroids*

A double-blind, randomised study compared the efficacy of twice-daily calcipotriol ointment with a combination of betamethasone dipropionate and salicylic acid ointment in 58 patients with nail psoriasis over 3 months [17]. Both treatments demonstrated similar levels of response in reducing subungual hyperkeratosis; however, only about half of the patients responded to treatment [17]. Rigopoulos et al. confirmed the benefits of using topical calcipotriol in combination with a topical steroid cream in an open-label study utilising calcipotriol cream on weekdays and clobetasol propionate at weekends over 6 months. This regimen produced a 77% reduction in subungual hyperkeratosis at 12-month follow-up [18]. A more recent study found that once-daily topical calcipot-

**Table 1.** Summary: topical treatments for nail psoriasis including level-of-evidence assignments as used by GRAPPA [17–21, 23, 24, 62–69]

| Authors, year | Number of patients studied | Trial type | Treatment protocol | Clinical result | Level of evidence |
|---|---|---|---|---|---|
| Baran R, Tosti A (1999) | Study A: 27 (26 completed) Study B: 18 (15 completed) | 2 × double-blind, placebo-controlled | 8% clobetasol-17-propionate nail lacquer applied to one hand; placebo lacquer applied to other hand. Study A: treatment applied once daily until end of treatment. Study B: treatment applied once daily in first week, 2–3 times weekly from second week onward. | Study A: 18 patients (69%) showed clear improvement after therapy; no response in 7 patients (27%); worsening in one patient (4%). Study B: 12 patients (80%) showed clear improvement after therapy; no response in 2 patients (13%); worsening in one patient (7%). | 2a |
| Bianchi L, Soda R, Diluvio L, Chimenti S (2003) | 35 (25 completed) | Randomised, open-label | Tazarotene 0.1% gel unoccluded applied at bedtime for 12 weeks | 19/25 showed good clinical response; statistically significant 'Visual Assessment Score' reduction for specific signs at 12 weeks ($p < 0.0001$) from baseline | 4 |
| Cannavo SP, Guarneri F, Vaccaro M, et al. (2003) | 16 (8 active treatment, 8 placebo) | Prospective, randomised, placebo-controlled | Oil solution containing 70% oral preparation ciclosporin and 30% maize oil or placebo (maize oil) applied to nails twice daily for 12 weeks | With active treatment, 3 patients came to complete resolution, 5 showed substantial improvement in overall severity score; with placebo, slight improvement was noted in one patient, minimal improvement in 3 patients and no changes in 4 patients. Mean improvement was 77% with active treatment and 12% with placebo (0–3 severity scores for each psoriatic nail feature). | 2b |
| De Jong EMGJ, Menke HE, van Praag MCG, van de Kerkhof PCM (1999) | 57 | Randomised, double-blind, left-right | 1% 5-fluorouracil in nail-penetrating enhancer formulation or vehicle applied once daily for 12 weeks | Both treatments produced statistically significant improvements; 1% 5-fluorouracil does not provide any additional efficacy. | 1b |
| Fredriksson T (1974) | 20 | Open | 1% 5-fluorouracil applied twice daily for 4–6 months | Severity of pitting and subungual hyperkeratosis improved by 75% in 17/20 subjects. | 4 |
| Kokelj F, Lavaroni G, Piraccini BM, Tosti A (1994) | 7 | Open-label | Topical calcipotriol 50 μg/g cream applied twice daily for 3 months | 5 patients experienced improvement of their nail psoriasis, one patient showed no improvement and one dropped out; after further treatment, complete clearing was observed in one patient. | 4 |
| Regana MS, Ezquerra GM, Millet PU, Mateos FL (2005) | 10 | Open | 8% clobetasol-17-propionate nail lacquer applied once daily for 21 days, then twice weekly for 9 months | 9 patients showed good clinical response; onycholysis, pitting and salmon patches showed best improvement; subungual hyperkeratosis showed moderate improvement; splinter haemorrhages seemed more persistent; nail pain disappeared after 4 weeks. | 4 |
| Rigopoulos D, Gregoriou S, Katsambas A (2007) | 46 (23 tazarotene, 16 completed; 23 clobetasol, 14 completed) | Randomised, double-blind | Either tazarotene 0.1% cream or clobetasol propionate 0.05% cream applied to affected nail plates, surrounding nail folds and periungual skin under occlusion at bedtime for 12 weeks | Significant time-effect improvement was shown for all 4 NAPSI parameters for both treatments. Comparison of the improvement between administered agents did not reach statistical significance. | 2b |

**Table 1** (continued)

| Authors, year | Number of patients studied | Trial type | Treatment protocol | Clinical result | Level of evidence |
|---|---|---|---|---|---|
| Rigopoulos D, Ioannides D, Prastitis N, Katsambas A (2002) | 62 (60 completed; 48 fingernails, 53 toenails) | Open-label | Calcipotriol cream every night, 5 times/week during weekdays; clobetasol propionate cream 2 times/week, on weekends for 6 months, then clobetasol propionate cream only 2 nights/week for 6 months | Reduction in mean thickness of hyperkeratosis: at 2 months, 35.2% fingernails, 32.6% toenails; at 6 months, 72.3% fingernails, 69.9% toenails; at 12 months, 81.2% fingernails, 72.5% toenails. | 4 |
| Scher RK, Stiller M, Zhu YI (2001) | 31 (21 tazarotene, 10 vehicle) | Double-blind, randomised, vehicle-controlled, parallel-group | Tazarotene 0.1% gel or vehicle gel applied to target fingernail and surrounding nail folds once daily, in the evening, for up to 24 weeks; one target nail was occluded, the other target nail was not | Tazarotene was consistently more effective than vehicle in reducing onycholysis in occluded nails and non-occluded nails at week 24; tazarotene was also more effective than vehicle in reducing pitting in occluded nails; all $p \leq 0.05$. No other significant differences. | 1b |
| Tosti A, Guerra L, Bardazzi F, Lanzarini M (1990) | 1 | Case report | 0.2 ml 10% oily solution ciclosporin once daily for 3 months | Pitting and onycholysis almost cleared. | 4 |
| Tosti A, Piraccini BM, Cameli N, et al. (1998) | 58–29 calcipotriol (23 completed), 29 betamethasone + salicylic acid (21 completed) | Double-blind, randomised, comparative | Either calcipotriol ointment (50 μg/g) or betamethasone dipropionate (64 mg/g) + salicylic acid (0.03 g/g) ointment was applied twice daily for 3 months (5 months for responders) | Fingernails: >50% reduction in subungual hyperkeratosis in at least one nail in 8/13 calcipotriol patients and 10/16 betamethasone + salicylic acid patients. Toenails: >50% reduction in subungual hyperkeratosis in at least one nail in 7/20 calcipotriol patients and 12/24 betamethasone + salicylic acid patients. No significant difference between treatments. | 2b |
| Tzung TY, Chen CY, Yang CY, et al. (2008) | 40 (32 completed) | Randomised, investigator-blind, actively controlled, parallel-group comparison | Group A: 0.005% calcipotriol + 0.05% betamethasone dipropionate ointment applied once daily for 12 weeks. Group B: 0.005% calcipotriol ointment applied twice daily for 12 weeks. | Compared with baseline, 53% of patients from either group showed at least moderate improvement after 12 weeks; reduction in NAPSI was noted for both treatments ($p \leq 0.45$). No significant difference between treatments. | 3 |
| Yamamoto T, Katayama I, Nishioka K (1998) | 20 | Open-label | 0.4%–2.0% anthralin in petroleum applied to affected nail bed once daily and washed away with water after 30 minutes; 10% triethanolamine cream was then applied to prevent undesired pigmentation. Concentration of anthralin was gradually increased from 0.4% to 2.0% if unresponsive. | After 5 months, 12 patients showed moderate and obvious improvement, 4 patients showed little improvement and 4 patients showed no response. | 4 |
| Zakeri M, Valikhani M, Mortazavi H, Barzegari M (2005) | 24 | Case series, open-label | Calcipotriol ointment (50 μg/g) applied without occlusion twice daily for 3 months (5 months for responders) | After 3 months, 14 patients showed significant improvement; 2 were completely free of nail lesions after 5 months. | 4 |

GRAPPA = Group for Research and Assessment of Psoriasis and Psoriatic Arthritis; NAPSI = Nail Psoriasis Severity Index.

riol and betamethasone dipropionate ointment was as effective as calcipotriol ointment applied twice daily in the treatment of nail psoriasis over 12 weeks [19]. Both topical treatments resulted in 53% of patients achieving at least a moderate improvement in investigator global assessment and a significant reduction in Nail Psoriasis Severity Index (NAPSI) score from baseline ($p < 0.05$) [19].

A case series study evaluating the efficacy and safety of calcipotriol ointment for the treatment of nail psoriasis in 24 patients found that calcipotriol was particularly effective in reducing hyperkeratosis, onycholysis and discolouration [20]. Following 3 months of therapy, 14 patients showed significant improvement, with 2 being completely free of nail lesions after 5 months [20]. After discontinuation of therapy, the majority of patients experienced recurrent lesions, although of lower severity [20].

*Other Topical Therapies*

Tazarotene 0.1% gel has been evaluated for the treatment of fingernail psoriasis in a double-blind, randomised, vehicle-controlled, parallel-group trial in 31 patients [21]. Although tazarotene was effective in reducing onycholysis and pitting, it had no significant effect on subungual hyperkeratosis, leuconychia, nail plate crumbling/loss, splinter haemorrhages or nail growth rate at 24 weeks [21]. Another double-blind, randomised study compared the efficacy of tazarotene cream with clobetasol propionate cream in nail psoriasis over a 12-week treatment period [22]. Of the 46 patients randomised (23 to each treatment), 14 did not complete the trial, largely due to a requirement for systemic medication as a result of cutaneous psoriasis deterioration. Both treatments were found to improve pitting, hyperkeratosis, onycholysis and salmon patches after 12 weeks ($p < 0.001$), although there was no statistically significant difference between the 2 treatments [22]. Lastly, an open study of tazarotene 0.1% gel demonstrated a good clinical response in 19 of 25 patients who completed the 12-week treatment protocol [23]. Nails were only visually assessed, with no standardised method of assessment used, and no occurrences of complete clearance were reported. However, recurrences were reported 24 weeks post treatment [23].

Another topical treatment, ciclosporin, can be applied in an oil solution and has demonstrated some efficacy in nail psoriasis in a prospective, randomised, placebo-controlled study [24]. All patients receiving ciclosporin ($n = 8$) showed improvement in nail severity score, with 3 patients achieving complete resolution after 12 weeks, compared with only one patient receiving placebo ($n = 8$) achieving a slight improvement [24].

*Intralesional Therapy*

Intralesional therapy is a conventional treatment option, despite the lack of randomised controlled trials or high-quality evidence. The therapy consists of injecting small doses of corticosteroid directly into or near the structure of the nail unit that is responsible for the specific nail dystrophy [25–29]. Although evidence is limited, intralesional injections appear to be particularly effective for alleviating lesions caused by psoriasis of the nail matrix, including certain nail plate abnormalities, such as pitting and ridging [1]. However, the use of intralesional therapy requires considerable motivation and tolerance by the patient, as it is a painful and tedious form of management [16].

Very little clinical data are available on the efficacy of intralesional injections, although many physicians consider this approach standard treatment for nail disease. De Berker and Lawrence conducted an open trial of intralesional steroid injections (triamcinolone 10 mg/ml) in 19 patients with nail psoriasis [25]. Onycholysis was improved in 50% of nails, pitting in 45%, transverse ridging in 93%, thickening in 83% and subungual hyperkeratosis in 100% [25]. However, complete resolution did not occur in all clinical manifestations, with only 20% of nails with pitting and only 25% with subungual hyperkeratosis reaching complete clearance [25].

The published evidence for intralesional treatment modalities in nail psoriasis is summarised in table 2.

*Phototherapy and Radiation Therapies*

Although the efficacy of phototherapy and photochemotherapy has been widely validated for treating skin psoriasis, there has been a clear absence of evidence regarding effects on nail psoriasis [1]. Psoralen plus ultraviolet A (PUVA) is one of the most common photochemotherapeutic regimens. The psoralen can be administered orally or topically, and at times, the nails can be soaked in the solution before exposure to ultraviolet A. PUVA appears to be successful in treating psoriasis arising from the nail bed (e.g., onycholysis, subungual hyperkeratosis) but does little to improve some nail matrix disease symptoms (e.g., pitting) [30, 31].

Superficial radiotherapy, a form of electromagnetic radiation, has proven to have some efficacy when treating nail psoriasis [32, 33], but the effect may be short-lived. Additional radiation therapies, such as Grenz ray therapy and electron beams, have both achieved a moderate im-

**Table 2.** Summary: intralesional therapies for nail psoriasis including level-of-evidence assignments as used by GRAPPA [25–29, 70]

| Authors, year | Number of patients studied | Trial type | Treatment protocol | Clinical result | Level of evidence |
|---|---|---|---|---|---|
| Abell E, Samman PD (1973) | 24 involving matrix only, 14 combined matrix and onycholysis, 14 psoriatic onycholysis | Open | Triamcinolone 5 mg/ml (1–4 injections of 0.1 ml/nail) injected with a needleless injector into the area of the fingernail matrix through the posterior nail fold on 3 occasions at 2–4 weekly intervals; severely dystrophic nails were subsequently given intermittent injections at 6–10 weekly intervals, as deemed necessary. | Matrix only: 19 normal/greatly improved, 2 improved, 3 no change. Combined matrix and onycholysis: result in matrix: 17 normal/greatly improved, 2 improved, 1 no change; result in onycholysis: 9 cleared/greatly improved, 5 improved, 6 no change. Psoriatic onycholysis: 3 cleared/greatly improved, 4 improved, 7 no change. | 4 |
| Bleeker JJ (1974) | 15 needleless injector, 18 conventional needle infiltration | Open, controlled | 3 × 0.2 ml triamcinolone 5 mg/ml infiltrated with needleless injector around the base of each nail 3–4 mm proximal to the nail plate; conventional needle infiltrations treating symmetrical lesions or 2 halves of same lesion: 0.1–0.2 ml triamcinolone 5 mg/ml infiltrated in each of 3 weals around the matrix. | Results were the same for needleless injector and conventional needle; needleless injector resulted in 80% success rate in healing 109 infiltrated nails. | 3 |
| De Berker DAR, Lawrence CM (1998) | 19 | Open-label | After anaesthetisation, triamcinolone acetonide 10 mg/ml was injected, 0.1 ml into each of 4 periungual sites. Further injection was offered at 2 months if poor response. | Onycholysis improved in 50%, pitting in 45%, subungual hyperkeratosis in 100%, transverse ridging in 94% and thickening in 83%. | 4 |
| Gerstein W (1962) | 4 | Case series | 0.2–0.25 ml of triamcinolone acetonide suspension 10 mg/ml injected into the matrix of involved fingernails after preliminary digital block anaesthesia with 0.5%–2% xylocaine | All patients showed a response: in only one nail in one patient. | 4 |
| Peachey RD, Pye RJ, Harman RR (1976) | 37 | Open | Using needleless injector, 1–3 deep intradermal injections of 0.1 ml of either triamcinolone acetonide (5 mg/ml) or triamcinolone hexacetonide (5 mg/ml) were given into the posterior nail fold of affected nails. | Pitting, ridging and other nail matrix changes improved in 90% of patients, while nail bed and/or hyponychial changes (mainly onycholysis) improved in only 26%. | 4 |
| Saleem K, Azim W (2008) | 35 | Open-label | Injection of triamcinolone acetonide (10 mg/ml) was given into the nail bed and matrix following ring block anaesthesia. Further injection was offered at 2 months if poor response. | Pitting improved in 57.7%, onycholysis in 40.5% and subungual hyperkeratosis in 70.1%. | 4 |

provement in nail psoriasis but are not commonly used to treat psoriasis [34, 35]. Furthermore, radiation therapy is associated with serious potential side effects, and it is often tedious and labourious; however, it may be useful for patients refractory to other, more convenient forms of treatment.

The published evidence for radiation and phototherapies in nail psoriasis is summarised in table 3.

### *Systemic Therapies*

Although conventional systemic therapies, such as ciclosporin, have been repeatedly shown to be effective in skin psoriasis, there is very little existing evidence that demonstrates their efficacy in improving nail disease [36]. A variety of systemic agents, including methotrexate, tacrolimus, sulphasalazine, azathioprine and calcitriol, have yet to be assessed with respect to nail disease.

**Table 3.** Summary: radiation and phototherapies for nail psoriasis including level-of-evidence assignments as used by GRAPPA [30–35]

| Authors, year | Number of patients studied | Trial type | Treatment protocol | Clinical result | Level of evidence |
|---|---|---|---|---|---|
| Finnerty EF (1979) | 3 | Case reports | Case 1: Superficial x-ray therapy, 8 treatments 75 r at 2-week intervals. Case 2: 8 treatments 75 r at 2-week intervals. Case 3: treatments of 50 r at weekly intervals, 300 r over 1 month. | Case 1: normal nails began to grow from bases – over 14 months, nails regrew normally. Case 2: nail regrowth was normal after 6 months. Case 3: much improvement after 15 weeks; after additional treatments, nails regrew normally. | 4 |
| Handfield-Jones SE, Boyle J, Harman RR (1987) | 5 | Open | 1% 8-methoxypsoralen solution applied to proximal nail fold up to the terminal phalanx, backs of hands exposed to UVA 3 mW/cm$^2$ at a distance of 20 cm: 0.5 increasing to 2 J max used 2–3 times/week | 2 patients cleared completely (later relapsed), 2 patients had no substantial improvement, one patient failed to show sustained improvement and ceased treatment. Onycholysis was more responsive than pitting. | 4 |
| Kwang TY, Nee TS, Seng KT (1995) | 12 | Open, controlled | Nails and beds of one hand treated with electron beam of 7 MeV; 8 fractions over 8 weeks (0.75 Gy/week); other hand used as control | 3 months after electron beam therapy, one patient showed marked improvement, 2 moderate improvement, 6 slight improvement and 3 failed to respond. Compared with control hand, statistically significant improvement at 3 months ($p < 0.05$) but not at 6 months ($p > 0.5$). | 2b |
| Lindelöf B (1989) | 24 (22 completed) | Double-blind, placebo-controlled | 5 Gy of Grenz rays on 10 occasions at intervals of 1 week; one hand active treatment, other hand placebo | Grenz ray-treated nails: one patient almost complete recovery, 7 slight improvement, 14 no improvement at all. Placebo-treated nails: one patient improved slightly. No hyperkeratotic nails responded. | 1b |
| Marx JL, Scher RK (1980) | 10 | Open | Methoxsalen 0.6 mg/kg given orally, 2 h later exposed to 320–400 nm of UVA radiation 9 mW/cm$^2$ 2–3 times/week | Of 26 involved nails, 18 improved by 50% or more; only pitting failed to respond in all 8 patients who had this change. | 4 |
| Yu RCH, King CM (1992) | 10 (8 completed) | Double-blind, controlled | Superficial radiotherapy administered to distal phalanx of randomly preselected hand: 3 fractionated doses of 150 cGy given at 2 weekly intervals; sham radiotherapy administered to other hand. | Significant clinical improvement at 10 and 15 weeks in radiotherapy-treated hands; significant reduction in nail thickness at 15 weeks; rate of nail growth not significantly reduced. Improvement was not sustained. | 1b |

UVA = Ultraviolet A.

Systemic therapy is often required in patients with nail psoriasis when extensive skin or joint disease is present or when topical therapies, intralesional therapies and phototherapies have failed [4]. Due to the potential toxicity of many systemic agents, they would not be recommended in patients presenting solely with nail disease [37].

The published evidence for systemic treatment modalities in nail psoriasis is summarised in table 4.

*Acitretin*

A recent open study involving 36 patients with moderate to severe psoriasis limited to the nails found that low-dose acitretin (0.2–0.3 mg/kg/day) produced a mean 41% reduction in the NAPSI score over 6 months [38]. For the most severely affected nail in each patient (target nail), there was a mean 50% reduction in modified NAPSI score [38]. After 6 months of treatment, 25% of patients were considered to show complete or almost complete

**Table 4.** Summary: systemic treatment for nail psoriasis including level-of-evidence assignments as used by GRAPPA [36–40, 71–75]

| Authors, year | Number of patients studied | Trial type | Treatment protocol | Clinical result | Level of evidence |
|---|---|---|---|---|---|
| Arnold WP, Gerritsen MJ, van de Kerkhof PC (1993) | 1 | Case report | Ciclosporin 3 mg/kg/day increased by 1 mg/kg/day when PASI >75% of the baseline value at weeks 4 and 8 | Substantial improvement in nail changes | 4 |
| Feliciani C, Zampetti A, Forleo P, et al. (2004) | 54 | Comparative, single-blinded (dermatologist) | All patients were treated with oral ciclosporin alone (3–4.5 mg/kg/day) divided into 2 administrations/day for 3 months; 33 patients also received topical calcipotriol 50 μg/g cream twice daily (with occlusive application at night). | After 3 months, improvement in nail lesions seen in 79% of patients receiving combination therapy and 47.6% of patients in ciclosporin monotherapy group. | 3 |
| Feuerman EJ, Nir MA (1973) | 16 (13 completed) | Double-blind, crossover | 100 mg allopurinol or placebo – 2 tablets 3 times daily for 8 weeks, followed by 8-week crossover to other treatment | No statistical difference in rate of nail growth | 3 |
| Gerster JC (2002) | 1 | Case report | Sulphasalazine 0.5 g daily increased to 2 g daily | Nail lesions receded and disappeared progressively | 4 |
| Lassus A (1997) | 30 patients overall (15 each group); 10 evaluable for nail changes in active treatment group (placebo not specified) | Randomised, double-blind | 10 ml colloidal silicic acid gel or placebo gel 3 times daily for 90 days taken orally; patients also applied gel topically to lesions on knees or elbows | 5/10 receiving active treatment showed complete cure of onychopathy after treatment | 1b |
| Levell NJ, Shuster S, Munro CS, Friedmann PS (1995) | 60 (30 each treatment group; 26 completed ciclosporin group, 24 dithranol group); with nail psoriasis: 13 in ciclosporin group (10 completed), 16 in dithranol group (15 completed) | Open, randomised, comparative | Oral ciclosporin as 2 daily doses of 2.5 mg/kg until 2 weeks after psoriasis cleared or dithranol (2–8% with 0.5% salicylic acid in emulsifying ointment) in conventional short-contact therapy administered on weekdays by clinic nursing staff and preceded by a sub-erythemal dose of UVB (at weekends, patients treated themselves at home). | With ciclosporin: 8 improved, one unchanged and one worsened.<br>With dithranol: 8 improved, 2 unchanged and 5 worsened. | 3 |
| Mahrle G, Schulze HJ, Färber L, et al. (1995) | 210 (66.5% had nail involvement) | Randomised | Ciclosporin 2.5 mg/kg/day or etretinate 0.5 mg/kg/day, which could be adjusted to 5.0 and 0.75 mg/kg/day, respectively, for 10 weeks; ciclosporin patients were then randomised to drug tapering over 12 weeks or topical dithranol; etretinate patients switched to topical dithranol. | Significant alleviation of nail involvement occurred in both groups but not during first 10 weeks. | 2b |
| Mrowietz U, Christophers E (1991) | 285 | Randomised, open, controlled | Ciclosporin 1.25 or 2.5 mg/kg/day increased up to 5 mg/kg/day in case of inadequate therapeutic effect | Nail involvement improved in all patients treated | 3 |
| Syuto T, Abe M, Ishibuchi H, Ishikawa O (2007) | 16 | Open-label | Ciclosporin 3.0 mg/kg/day twice daily before meals; in patients whose nails improved, dose was reduced to 1.5 mg/kg/day in a single administration before breakfast | 15/16 patients showed improvement: 2 complete resolution, 10 significant improvement, 3 slight improvement, one patient no change | 4 |
| Tosti A, Ricotti C, Romanelli P, et al. (2009) | 36 | Open-label | Acitretin 0.2–0.3 mg/kg/day for 6 months | Mean reduction in NAPSI score 41%; 50% reduction in mean modified NAPSI for target nail.<br>At 6 months, complete or almost complete clearing in 9 patients (25%), moderate improvement in 9 patients (25%), mild improvement in 12 patients (33%) and no improvement in 6 patients (11%). | 4 |

PASI = Psoriasis Area and Severity Index; UVB = ultraviolet B.

clearance of nail lesions, with moderate improvement in a further 25% and mild improvement in 33%; however, 11% showed no improvement [38].

*Ciclosporin*

Some evidence for the efficacy of low-dose ciclosporin in the treatment of nail psoriasis has been provided by a small uncontrolled trial in 16 patients, 13 of whom were unresponsive to previous treatment [39]. Most patients (15/16) showed at least a slight improvement, with 2 patients achieving complete resolution and 10 demonstrating significant improvement [39].

The efficacy of systemic ciclosporin has been shown to be enhanced by the application of topical calcipotriol cream in a comparative single-blinded study of 54 patients (33 patients received ciclosporin alone, and 21 also applied calcipotriol cream) [40]. After 3 months of combination treatment, 79% of patients were reported to have a good or excellent level of improvement compared with 48% of those receiving ciclosporin alone [40].

## The Advent of New Treatment Options with Biologic Therapy

Conventional therapies for nail psoriasis have proven at times to be both painful and inconvenient for the patient, and most achieve only moderate efficacy for specific clinical manifestations of the nail disease. Recently, biologic agents, such as those targeted against tumour necrosis factor (TNF), have been employed to treat both cutaneous and nail psoriasis as well as PsA. With the increasing use of biologic therapy for the skin and with joint manifestations of psoriasis becoming more common, reports of efficacy in nail psoriasis are likely to become prevalent. Although there are presently few controlled studies of biologic therapy for nail psoriasis, many are in progress [6].

The published evidence for biologic treatment modalities in nail psoriasis is summarised in table 5. A further review of the published randomised, double-blind, placebo-controlled trials is presented in table 6.

*Adalimumab*

Adalimumab, a TNF inhibitor given by subcutaneous injection (40 mg) every 2 weeks, demonstrated a clinically significant improvement in NAPSI score after 12 weeks of treatment in patients with active PsA and nail psoriasis (n = 259) in a large, open-label, prospective study [41]. An approximate 45% decrease in the mean NAPSI score was demonstrated by week 12 and continued, with a 65% decrease by week 20. Improvements in NAPSI score were independent of the magnitude of changes in other skin assessment measures and occurred regardless of joint response status [41].

*Alefacept*

Alefacept, a T-cell activation inhibitor, has demonstrated limited response in nail psoriasis. In an open-label prospective study, 449 patients with chronic plaque psoriasis were treated with up to 3 courses of intramuscular alefacept. Some level of improvement in at least one nail was observed in 57–71% of patients who had nail disease at baseline [42]. However, only 13–20% of patients exhibited improvement in all involved nails from baseline, and the magnitude of improvement was not defined [42].

Additional small clinical studies have been completed with alefacept that support a poor to moderate response in nail psoriasis with demonstrated equivocal results for nail symptoms [43–45].

*Etanercept*

Etanercept, a TNF inhibitor, has shown efficacy in nail psoriasis in an open-label, randomised trial (CRYSTEL) including 564 patients with moderate to severe psoriasis with nail involvement receiving etanercept for 54 weeks, either continuously or in a paused treat-to-response fashion [12]. Mean NAPSI scores decreased by 28.9% at 12 weeks ($p < 0.001$) and continued to decrease by 51% at 54 weeks [12]. Furthermore, at the end of treatment, 30% of patients with nail psoriasis at baseline reported complete clearance [12].

A double-blind, randomised, placebo-controlled trial in adolescents and children with moderate to severe psoriasis and nail involvement (n = 34) receiving continuous etanercept (n = 12) or placebo (n = 22) showed a 36% decrease in NAPSI score at week 12 with etanercept compared with only 0.1% for those receiving placebo [46]. Open-label treatment was then provided to all patients for the next 24 weeks, and the mean percentage reduction in NAPSI score from baseline was 47% for patients receiving etanercept for 36 weeks and 67% for patients initially receiving placebo followed by 24 weeks of etanercept treatment [46].

*Ustekinumab*

Ustekinumab, an anti-interleukin-12/23p40 monoclonal antibody, has been investigated in a double-blind, placebo-controlled trial of patients with moderate to severe psoriasis [47]. In the 545 patients with nail involvement at baseline, those receiving ustekinumab achieved a me-

**Table 5.** Summary: biologic therapies for nail psoriasis including level-of-evidence assignments as used by GRAPPA [12, 43–45, 48–52]

| Authors, year | Number of patients studied | Trial type | Treatment protocol | Clinical result | Level of evidence |
|---|---|---|---|---|---|
| Bianchi L, Bergamin A, de Felice C, et al. (2005) | 25 | Open | Infliximab 5 mg/kg at weeks 0, 2, 6, 14 and 22 | At week 14, all patients had shown at least a 50% reduction in NAPSI score from baseline. At week 22, mean NAPSI was 0 ($p < 0.0001$) – clinical remission in all patients. | 4 |
| Carr D, Tusa MG, Carroll CL, et al. (2008) | 15 (14 completed) | Open | Alefacept 15 mg/week IM for 16 weeks; increased to 30 mg/week at week 9 if palmoplantar pustular psoriasis not responding | Nail severity scores significantly improved ($p = 0.0003$) from baseline at week 28 | 4 |
| Hussain W, Coulson I, Owen C (2008) | 2 | Case report | Infliximab 5 mg/kg at weeks 0, 2 and 6 | Patient 1: after third infusion, NAPSI fell from 24 at baseline to 3. Patient 2: after single infusion, NAPSI fell from 22 to 6. | 4 |
| Korver JEM, Langewouters AMG, Van de Kerkhof PCM, Pasch MC (2006) | 8 | Open, prospective | Alefacept 15 mg/week IM for 12 weeks | Patients with initial NAPSI >15 (n = 5): 2 showed improvement, 2 unchanged, one nail pathology aggravated. Patients with initial NAPSI ≤15 (n = 3): one patient improved, one no change, one nail changes worsened. | 4 |
| Luger TA, Barker J, Lambert J, et al. (2009) | 564 | Randomised, open-label | Etanercept 25 mg SC twice weekly for 54 weeks (continuous) or 50 mg SC twice weekly for maximum of 12 weeks until psoriasis response, then stopped, and reinitiated at 25 mg SC twice weekly in the event of relapse (paused) – treat-to-target cycle continued throughout study | For all patients, at week 12, NAPSI improved by 28.9% ($p < 0.001$); at week 54, NAPSI improved by 51%; 30% of patients clear of nail disease at week 54 | 4 |
| Parrish CA, Sobera JO, Robbins CM, et al. (2006) | 15 | Prospective, open-label, proof-of-concept | Alefacept 15 mg IM every week for 12 weeks | At 24 weeks, mean NAPSI reduction from baseline was 39% ($p = 0.0002$): 53% reduction in nail matrix disease score ($p \leq 0.0001$) and 20% reduction in nail bed disease score ($p = 0.0952$) | 4 |
| Rich P, Griffiths CEM, Reich K, et al. (2008) Also: Reich K, Nestle FO, Papp K, et al. (2005) | 305 (65 placebo, 240 infliximab) | Double-blind, placebo-controlled, randomised | Infliximab 5 mg/kg or placebo IV infusions at weeks 0, 2 and 6 and every 8 weeks thereafter. Patients receiving placebo crossed over to infliximab at weeks 24, 26 and 30 and every 8 weeks through week 46 in a double-blind fashion. | At weeks 10 and 24, the percentage reduction from baseline of the NAPSI was significantly greater in infliximab-treated patients than placebo-treated patients (26.8 vs. –7.7% at week 10; 57.2 vs. –4.1% at week 24; $p < 0.001$ both comparisons). At week 50, mean improvement in NAPSI score from baseline was 59.7% for those receiving infliximab throughout. | 1b |
| Rigopoulos D, Gregoriou S, Stratigos A, et al. (2008) | 18 | Open, non-randomised, non-blinded | Infliximab 5 mg/kg infusions at baseline, 2 weeks, 6 weeks and every 8 weeks thereafter | At week 14, significant reductions in mean NAPSI were seen (55.8 at baseline, 29.8 at week 14); at week 38, there was almost complete resolution of psoriatic nail involvement (mean NAPSI 3.3) | 4 |

dian 25% improvement in NAPSI score at week 12 compared with 0% for those receiving placebo. Nail psoriasis continued to improve in patients in all groups treated with ustekinumab over time after the placebo-controlled portion of the study, and improvements were sustained through 1 year [47].

*Infliximab*

Several trials and case reports have demonstrated that infliximab, a TNF inhibitor administered intravenously, provides significant improvement in patients with moderate to severe psoriasis with nail involvement [48–51].

**Table 6.** Randomised, double-blind, placebo-controlled trials of biologic therapy in nail psoriasis [46–48]

| Trial | Subjects | Therapy | Outcome measure | Results |
|---|---|---|---|---|
| Pariser D et al. [Pariser EADV, 2008] | 34 moderate to severe psoriasis patients aged 4–17 years | Etanercept 0.8 mg/kg (n = 12) or placebo (n = 22) for 12 weeks | NAPSI | At 12 weeks, etanercept reduced mean NAPSI score by 36% compared with 0.1% placebo |
| PHOENIX 1 Rich P et al. [Rich AAD, 2008] | 545 moderate to severe psoriasis patients aged ≥18 years | Ustekinumab 45 mg (n = 182) or 90 mg (n = 187) or placebo (n = 176) at weeks 0 and 4 | NAPSI, nail PGA | At 12 weeks, the median NAPSI score was reduced by 25% in both ustekinumab groups compared with 0% placebo.<br>A nail PGA score of none or mild was achieved in 69.8% ustekinumab 45 mg patients, 71.7% ustekinumab 90 mg patients and 48.9% placebo patients at 12 weeks. |
| EXPRESS Rich P et al. [Rich, 2008] | 305 moderate to severe psoriasis patients aged ≥18 years | Infliximab 5 mg/kg (n = 240) or placebo (n = 65) at weeks 0, 2, 6, 14 and 22 | NAPSI | At week 10, mean percent NAPSI improvement was 26.8% with infliximab and –7.7% with placebo.<br>At week 24, mean percent NAPSI improvement was 57.2% with infliximab and –4.1% with placebo. |

PGA = Physician's Global Assessment.

In a large phase III, multicentre, double-blind, placebo-controlled study (EXPRESS) designed to evaluate the efficacy and safety of infliximab in patients with moderate to severe psoriasis, patients received 5 mg/kg at weeks 0, 2 and 6, followed by infusion every 8 weeks [52]. Rich et al. subsequently analysed the data and demonstrated that of 305 patients with moderate to severe psoriasis and nail involvement, improvement was demonstrated from week 10, with complete clearance of the target nail in almost half of patients (44.7%) at 1 year [48]. Mean percentage improvements in NAPSI score at weeks 10 and 24 were 26.8 and 57.2%, respectively, in the infliximab group versus –7.7 and –4.1%, respectively, in the placebo group [48]. More than two thirds of patients demonstrated resolution of some nail bed and matrix manifestations by week 10.

Two small studies also support the efficacy of infliximab in the treatment of nail psoriasis. An unblinded, non-randomised, open-label study of infliximab in 18 patients with nail psoriasis noted significant improvement in NAPSI scores after the third infusion of infliximab (week 14) [51]. A 47% reduction in mean NAPSI score was evident at week 14, and at week 38 (after 6 infusions), a 94% reduction in mean NAPSI score was evident, representing almost complete resolution of psoriatic nail involvement [51]. In another open-label, prospective study of 25 patients presenting with severe onychodystrophy, infliximab demonstrated the ability to completely clear nail disease (mean NAPSI = 0) in all patients at 22 weeks [49]. Furthermore, during a follow-up period of 12 weeks from the last infusion, patients maintained their clinical remission of nail psoriasis [49]. Infliximab is the only biologic agent to have demonstrated complete clearance of nail disease in a high proportion of patients in clinical studies. Examples of the use of infliximab in nail psoriasis can be seen in figure 1.

### *Comparison of TNF Inhibitors*

Recently, a prospective study allocated TNF inhibitor treatment for psoriasis or PsA with severe nail involvement (NAPSI >14) to 42 consecutive patients: 14 patients received adalimumab, 14 received etanercept and 14 received infliximab [53]. At week 6, there was a 28% reduction in NAPSI score in the adalimumab-treated group, 56% in the etanercept-treated group and 63% in the infliximab-treated group. Infliximab was the only agent to achieve a significant reduction in NAPSI score at week 6 ($p < 0.001$). Adalimumab and etanercept failed to achieve significant reductions in NAPSI score until the week 22 evaluation. At week 22, the NAPSI score reductions were 65% ($p < 0.001$), 64% ($p < 0.005$) and 89% ($p < 0.001$) for adalimumab, etanercept and infliximab, respectively. These results suggest that infliximab is more efficacious for nail symptoms in psoriasis than either adalimumab or etanercept and that it has a more rapid onset of action.

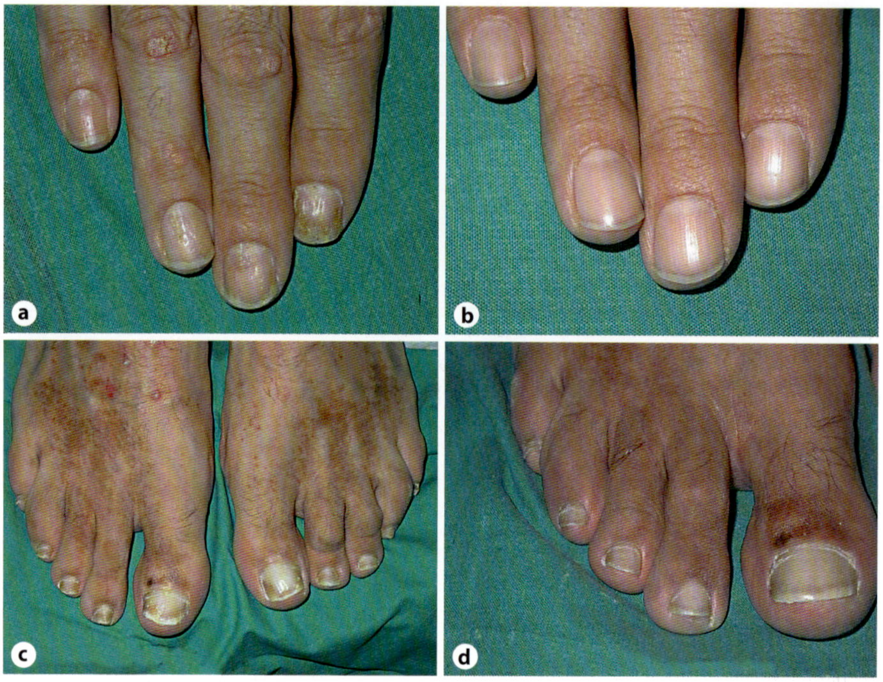


**Fig. 1.** Infliximab nail treatment response. **a** Fingernail psoriasis at baseline. **b** Fingernail psoriasis after 6th infliximab infusion. **c** Toenail psoriasis at baseline. **d** Toenail psoriasis after 6th infliximab infusion.

## Evidence-Based Treatment of Cutaneous and Nail Psoriasis with Biologic Agents

Awareness is increasing that psoriasis as a disease is more than just cutaneous symptoms; the nails and joints can also be affected, with considerable impact on patient quality of life [5, 6, 9, 12]. Furthermore, nail involvement in psoriasis may be predictive of a more severe disease course and an indicator of the potential for joint involvement. Early intervention could provide the possibility of inducing remission in such patients before function and quality of life are even more severely affected [5, 6, 9, 54].

Based on current evidence (tables 5 and 6), TNF inhibitors are the most effective biologic agents for the treatment of nail psoriasis. The efficacy of TNF inhibitors in the treatment of both plaque psoriasis and PsA is also well established [55–57]. Indeed, use of TNF inhibitors has been associated with complete clearance of both skin and nail disease [48, 49, 58]. Clearance of psoriatic skin disease, as demonstrated by Psoriasis Area and Severity Index (PASI) responses, is known to correlate with patient-reported improvement in quality of life [59]. Biologics may be safer and more effective than traditional systemic therapies, based on outcomes from studies with retinoids, ciclosporin, methotrexate and PUVA [4].

Given that psoriatic nail disease often co-exists with PsA and may even be a precursor to distal interphalangeal joint involvement, treatment with the potential to prevent radiographic progression of PsA should be of benefit to patients who may have subclinical or undiagnosed disease, as well as those already diagnosed with PsA [55–57, 60]. The recent Group for Research and Assessment of Psoriasis and Psoriatic Arthritis (GRAPPA) treatment recommendations for PsA state that 'the efficacy of therapies for psoriatic nail disease is not well studied' [61]. Recommendations by GRAPPA for treatment of nail disease include retinoids, PUVA, ciclosporin and infliximab [61]. TNF inhibitors are also recommended, based on available evidence, for moderate to severe peripheral arthritis, moderate to severe skin disease and moderate to severe spinal disease [61]. For severe enthesitis, infliximab and etanercept are specified as having evidence for use, while in dactylitis, infliximab is the only biologic agent recommended and has the highest level of evidence [61].

## Conclusions

Nail psoriasis is often overlooked by physicians and, importantly, is not included in measures of cutaneous severity, such as the PASI. However, nail psoriasis can have a significant impact on patient quality of life, causing significant physical impairment and pain. Nail psoriasis may also be closely linked to PsA, providing a link to the diagnosis of this progressive disabling condition. The options for treating nail psoriasis are much more limited in scope than those for skin disease. Many are not proven in controlled clinical trials and are tedious and sometimes painful to administer, and their effects are short-lived. Biologic therapies are showing promise in the treatment of nail psoriasis, and although randomised, placebo-controlled trials are currently sparse, the evidence base is growing. The TNF inhibitor infliximab appears to have the most robust clinical data set supporting its use as an effective treatment for nail psoriasis. Use of infliximab has been shown to result in complete clearance of nail disease with maintained remission and to provide improvements in patient quality of life.

In general, when assessing the psoriasis patient, a holistic approach considering not only the cutaneous manifestations, but also the nail and possible joint symptoms, should help inform treatment decisions to ensure that the impact on the patient's life is minimised.

## Conflicts of Interest

Richard Langley and Estaban Daudén serve as investigators, scientific speakers and consultants for Schering Corporation, a subsidiary of Merck & Co., Inc. Dr. Langley has also served as a principal investigator or scientific advisor for Merck-Serono, Abbott, Amgen, Johnson & Johnson, Pfizer, and Boehringer Ingelheim. Editorial support for the development of this publication was provided by Schering Corporation, a subsidiary of Merck & Co., Inc.

## References


1 Jiaravuthisan MM, Sasseville D, Vender RB, Murphy F, Muhn CY: Psoriasis of the nail: anatomy, pathology, clinical presentation, and a review of the literature on therapy. J Am Acad Dermatol 2007;57:1–27.

2 Sanchez-Regna M, Umbert P: Diagnosis and management of nail psoriasis. Actas Dermosifiliogr 2008;99:34–43.

3 Samman PD, Fenton DA: The Nails in Disease, ed 5. London, Butterworth-Heinemann Ltd., 1994.

4 Gregoriou S, Kalogeromitros D, Kosionis N, Gkouvi A, Rigopoulos D: Treatment options for nail psoriasis. Expert Rev Dermatol 2008; 3:339–344.

5 Williamson L, Dalbeth N, Dockerty JL, Gee BC, Weatherall R, Wordsworth BP: Extended report: nail disease in psoriatic arthritis – clinically important, potentially treatable and often overlooked. Rheumatology (Oxford) 2004;43:790–794.

6 Lawry M: Biological therapy and nail psoriasis. Dermatol Ther 2007;20:60–67.

7 De Jong EMGJ, Seegers BAMPA, Gulinck MK, Boezeman JBM, van de Kerkhof PCM: Psoriasis of the nails associated with disability in a large number of patients: results of a recent interview with 1,728 patients. Dermatology 1996;193:300–303.

8 Helliwell P, Marchesoni A, Peters M, Barker M, Wright V: A re-evaluation of the osteoarticular manifestations of psoriasis. Br J Rheumatol 1991;30:339–345.

9 Landells I, MacCallum C, Khraishi M: The role of the dermatologist in identification and treatment of the early stages of psoriatic arthritis. Skin Therapy Lett 2008;13:4–8.

10 Salomon J, Szepietowski JC, Proniewicz A: Psoriatic nails: a prospective clinical study. J Cutan Med Surg 2003;7:317–321.

11 Wilson FC, Icen M, Crowson CS, et al: Incidence and clinical predictors of psoriatic arthritis in patients with psoriasis: a population-based study. Arthritis Rheum 2009;61: 233–239.

12 Luger TA, Barker J, Lambert J, et al: Sustained improvement in joint pain and nail symptoms with etanercept therapy in patients with moderate-to-severe psoriasis. J Eur Acad Dermatol Venereol 2009;23:896–904.

13 Guero S, Guichard S, Fraitag SR: Ligamentary structure of the base of the nail. Surg Radiol Anat 1994;16:47–52.

14 Tan AL, Benjamin M, Toumi H, Grainger AJ, Tanner SF, Emery P, McGonagle D: The relationship between the extensor tendon enthesis and the nail in distal interphalangeal joint disease in psoriatic arthritis – a high-resolution MRI and histological study. Rheumatology (Oxford) 2007;46:253–256.

15 Baran R, Dawber RPR (eds): Diseases of the Nail and Their Management. Oxford, Blackwell Science, 1984.

16 De Berker DAR: Management of nail psoriasis. Clin Exp Dermatol 2000;25:357–362.

17 Tosti A, Piraccini BM, Cameli N, et al: Calcipotriol ointment in nail psoriasis: a controlled double-blind comparison with betamethasone dipropionate and salicylic acid. Br J Dermatol 1998;139:655–659.

18 Rigopoulos D, Ioannides D, Prastitis N, Katsambas A: Nail psoriasis: a combined treatment using calcipotriol cream and clobetasol propionate cream. Acta Derm Venereol 2002;82:140.

19 Tzung TY, Chen CY, Yang CY, et al: Calcipotriol used as monotherapy or combination therapy with betamethasone dipropionate in the treatment of nail psoriasis. Acta Derm Venereol 2008;88:279–280.

20 Zakeri M, Valikhani M, Mortazavi H, Barzegari M: Topical calcipotriol therapy in nail psoriasis: a study of 24 cases. Dermatol Online J 2005;11:5.

21 Scher RK, Stiller M, Zhu YI: Tazarotene 0.1% gel in the treatment of fingernail psoriasis: a double-blind, randomized, vehicle-controlled study. Cutis 2001;68:355–358.

22 Rigopoulos D, Gregoriou S, Katsambas A: Treatment of psoriatic nails with tazarotene cream 0.1% vs. clobetasol propionate 0.05% cream: a double-blind study. Acta Derm Venereol 2007;87:167–189.

23 Bianchi L, Soda R, Diluvio L, Chimenti S: Tazarotene 0.1% gel for psoriasis of the fingernails and toenails: an open, prospective study. Br J Dermatol 2003;149:207–209.

24 Cannavo SP, Guarneri F, Vaccaro M, Borgia F, Guarneri B: Treatment of psoriatic nails with topical cyclosporine: a prospective, randomized placebo-controlled study. Dermatology 2003;206:152–156.

25 De Berker DAR, Lawrence CM: A simplified protocol of steroid injection for psoriatic nail dystrophy. Br J Dermatol 1998;138:90–95.

26 Gerstein W: Psoriasis and lichen planus of nails. Treatment with triamcinolone. Arch Dermatol 1962;86:419–421.

27 Abell E, Samman PD: Intradermal triamcinolone treatment of nail dystrophies. Br J Dermatol 1973;89:191–197.

28 Bleeker JJ: Intralesional triamcinolone acetonide using the Port-O-Jet and needle injections in localized dermatoses. Br J Dermatol 1974;91:97–101.

29 Peachey RD, Pye RJ, Harman RR: The treatment of psoriatic nail dystrophy with intradermal steroid injections. Br J Dermatol 1976;95:75–78.

30 Marx JL, Scher RK: Response of psoriatic nails to oral photochemotherapy. Arch Dermatol 1980;116:1023–1024.
31 Handfield-Jones SE, Boyle J, Harman RR: Local PUVA treatment for nail psoriasis. Br J Dermatol 1987;116:280–281.
32 Yu RCH, King CM: A double-blind study of superficial radiotherapy in psoriatic nail dystrophy. Acta Derm Venereol 1992;72: 134–136.
33 Finnerty EF: Successful treatment of psoriasis of the nails. Cutis 1979;23:43–44.
34 Lindelöf B: Psoriasis of the nails treated with Grenz rays: a double-blind bilateral trial. Acta Derm Venereol 1989;69:80–82.
35 Kwang TY, Nee TS, Seng KT: A therapeutic study of nail psoriasis using electron beams. Acta Derm Venereol 1995;75:90.
36 Levell NJ, Shuster S, Munro CS, Friedmann PS: Remission of ordinary psoriasis following a short clearance course of cyclosporin. Acta Derm Venereol 1995;75:65–69.
37 Mahrle G, Schulze HJ, Färber L, Weidinger G, Steigleder GK: Low-dose short-term cyclosporine versus etretinate in psoriasis: improvement of skin, nail, and joint involvement. J Am Acad Dermatol 1995;32:78–88.
38 Tosti A, Ricotti C, Romanelli P, et al: Evaluation of the efficacy of acitretin therapy for nail psoriasis. Arch Dermatol 2009;145:269–271.
39 Syuto T, Abe M, Ishibuchi H, Ishikawa O: Successful treatment of psoriatic nails with low-dose cyclosporine administration. Eur J Dermatol 2007;17:248–249.
40 Feliciani C, Zampetti A, Forleo P, et al: Nail psoriasis: combined therapy with systemic cyclosporine and topical calcipotriol. J Cutan Med Surg 2004;8:122–125.
41 Van den Bosch F, Reece R, Behrens F, et al: Clinically important nail psoriasis improvements are achieved with adalimumab (Humira®): results from a large open-label prospective study (STEREO). Ann Rheum Dis 2007;66(suppl II):421.
42 Korman N, Rico MJ: Multiple courses of alefacept for the treatment of psoriatic nail disease in patients with chronic plaque psoriasis. J Am Acad Dermatol 2007;56:AB114, P1510.
43 Korver JEM, Langewouters AMG, Van de Kerkhof PCM, Pasch MC: Therapeutic effects of a 12-week course of alefacept on nail psoriasis. J Eur Acad Dermatol Venereol 2006;20:1252–1255.
44 Carr D, Tusa MG, Carroll CL, et al: Open label trial of alefacept in palmoplantar pustular psoriasis. J Dermatol Treat 2008;19:97–100.
45 Parrish CA, Sobera JO, Robbins CM, et al: Alefacept in the treatment of psoriatic nail disease: a proof of concept study. J Drugs Dermatol 2006;5:339–340.
46 Pariser D, Paller AS, Sigfried E, et al: Effect of etanercept treatment on skin and nail psoriasis symptoms in children and adolescents. EADV 2008, poster P448.
47 Rich P, Guzzo C, Wang Y, Gordon K: Improvement in nail psoriasis with ustekinumab, a new anti-IL-12/23p40 monoclonal antibody: results from a phase 3 trial. AAD 2008.
48 Rich P, Griffiths CEM, Reich K, et al: Baseline nail disease in patients with moderate to severe psoriasis and response to treatment with infliximab during 1 year. J Am Acad Dermatol 2008;58:224–231.
49 Bianchi L, Bergamin A, de Felice C, Capriotti E, Chimenti S: Remission and time of resolution of nail psoriasis during infliximab therapy. J Am Acad Dermatol 2005;52: 736–737.
50 Hussain W, Coulson I, Owen C: Severe recalcitrant nail psoriasis responding dramatically to infliximab: report of two patients. Clin Exp Dermatol 2008;33:520–522.
51 Rigopoulos D, Gregoriou S, Stratigos A, et al: Evaluation of the efficacy and safety of infliximab on psoriatic nails: an unblinded, nonrandomized, open-label study. Br J Dermatol 2008;159:453–456.
52 Reich K, Nestle FO, Papp K, et al: Infliximab induction and maintenance therapy for moderate-to-severe psoriasis: a phase III, multicentre, double-blind trial. Lancet 2005; 366:1367–1374.
53 Saraceno R, Bianchi L, Pietroleonardo L, et al: Remission and time of resolution of nail psoriasis: a comparison among antitumour necrosis factor-alpha inhibitors. Br J Dermatol 2008;159:1418, P47.
54 Gudjonsson JE, Karason A, Runarsdottir EH, et al: Distinct clinical differences between HLA-Cw*0602 positive and negative psoriasis patients – an analysis of 1019 HLA-C- and HLA-B-typed patients. J Invest Dermatol 2006;126:740–745.
55 Enbrel Summary of Product Characteristics (SPC).
56 Abbott Laboratories Limited: Humira pen and syringe. Summary of product characteristics. September 2008.
57 Schering-Plough Ltd: Remicade 100 mg powder for concentrate for solution for infusion. Summary of product characteristics. August 2008.
58 Rallis E, Stavropoulou E, Rigopoulos D, Verros C: Rapid response of nail psoriasis to etanercept. J Rheumatol 2008;35:544–545.
59 Reich K, Griffiths CEM: The relationship between quality of life and skin clearance in moderate-to-severe psoriasis: lessons learnt from clinical trials with infliximab. Arch Dermatol Res 2008;300:537–544.
60 Kavanaugh A, Antoni CE, Gladman D, et al: The infliximab multinational psoriatic arthritis controlled trial (IMPACT): results of radiographic analyses after 1 year. Ann Rheum Dis 2006;65:1038–1043.
61 Ritchlin CT, Kavanaugh A, Gladman DD, et al: Treatment recommendations for psoriatic arthritis. Ann Rheum Dis 2009;68:1387–1394.
62 Baran R, Tosti A: Topical treatment of nail psoriasis with a new corticoid-containing nail lacquer formulation. J Dermatol Treat 1999;10:201–204.
63 De Jong EMGJ, Menke HE, van Praag MCG, van de Kerkhof PCM: Dystrophic psoriatic fingernails treated with 1% 5-fluorouracil in a nail penetration-enhancing vehicle: a double-blind study. Dermatology 1999;199:313–318.
64 Fredriksson T: Topically applied fluorouracil in the treatment of psoriatic nails. Arch Dermatol 1974;110:735–736.
65 Kokelj F, Lavaroni G, Piraccini BM, Tosti A: Nail psoriasis treated with calcipotriol (MC 903): an open study. J Dermatol Treat 1994;5: 149–150.
66 Rigopoulos D, Gregoriou S, Katsambas A: Treatment of psoriatic nails with tazarotene cream 0.1% vs. clobetasol propionate 0.05% cream: a double-blind study. Acta Derm Venereol 2007;87:167–189.
67 Regana MS, Ezquerra GM, Millet PU, Mateos FL: Treatment of nail psoriasis with 8% clobetasol nail lacquer: positive experience in 10 patients. J Eur Acad Dermatol Venereol 2005;19:573–577.
68 Tosti A, Guerra L, Bardazzi F, Lanzarini M: Topical ciclosporin in nail psoriasis. Dermatologica 1990;180:110.
69 Yamamoto T, Katayama I, Nishioka K: Topical anthralin therapy for refractory nail psoriasis. J Dermatol 1998;25:231–233.
70 Saleem K, Azim W: Treatment of nail psoriasis with a modified regimen of steroid injections. J Coll Physicians Surg Pak 2008;18: 78–81.
71 Arnold WP, Gerritsen MJ, van de Kerkhof PC: Response of nail psoriasis to cyclosporin. Br J Dermatol 1993;129:750–751.
72 Feuerman EJ, Nir MA: Allopurinol in psoriasis – a double-blind study. Br J Dermatol 1973;89:83–86.
73 Gerster JC: Nail lesions in psoriatic arthritis: recovery with sulfasalazine treatment. Ann Rheum Dis 2002;61:277.
74 Lassus A: Colloidal silicic acid for the treatment of psoriatic skin lesions, arthropathy and onychopathy: a pilot study. J Int Med Res 1997;25:206–209.
75 Mrowietz U, Christophers E: Low-dose ciclosporin A (Sandimmun®) in psoriasis: a multicenter dose-finding study. Z Hautkr 1991;66(suppl 1):25–29.

Dermatology

Dermatology 2010;221(suppl 1):43–47
DOI: 10.1159/000316184

Published online: August 9, 2010

# The Impact of Methodological Approaches for Presenting Long-Term Clinical Data on Estimates of Efficacy in Psoriasis Illustrated by Three-Year Treatment Data on Infliximab

M. Papoutsaki[a] M. Talamonti[b] A. Giunta[b] A. Costanzo[b] M. Ruzzetti[b] M. Teoli[b] S. Chimenti[b]

[a]Third Department of Dermatology, A. Sygros Hospital, Athens, Greece; [b]Department of Dermatology, University of Rome Tor Vergata, Rome, Italy

**Key Words**

Plaque-type psoriasis · Infliximab · Long-term data · Analytical methodology

**Abstract**

***Background:*** Psoriasis affects about 2–3% of the Caucasian population. Biologics such as infliximab, etanercept, adalimumab and ustekinumab are efficacious treatments of plaque-type psoriasis. Critical to monitoring drug efficacy and safety is availability of long-term data. Despite the chronic nature of psoriasis, to date limited long-term clinical data have been available, as challenges are inherent in conducting a long-term analysis. With increasing time, it is more likely that the number of patients discontinuing treatment will also increase, due to loss of efficacy, adverse events or loss to follow-up. Interpretation of these data becomes confounded when one must consider missing data. Several approaches to analysing long-term data exist, and each accounts for missing data differently. ***Objective:*** To demonstrate that the choice of a particular analysis method to account for missing data has great impact on the assessed response rate. ***Methods:*** We used data from an open-label study over 3 years of continuous treatment with infliximab in patients with plaque-type psoriasis. These data were analysed by three methods – last observation carried forward, observed values and non-responder imputation – to account for missing data. ***Results:*** The 3-year PASI 75 responses varied from 41 to 75%, depending on the method of analysis; this shows that the response rate can almost double when a more liberal analytical approach is used. ***Conclusions:*** While it is clear that the need for long-term data on biologics in psoriasis is great, considering the analysis undertaken is important when designing long-term studies and interpreting the resulting data. When analysis methods such as observed values only or last observation carried forward are used, the results of the more conservative non-responder imputation should also be presented to give a fair overview of the long-term efficacy of a treatment for plaque-type psoriasis.



## Introduction

Psoriasis is a chronic papulosquamous skin disease [1] affecting approximately 2–3% of the Caucasian population [2]. Plaque-type psoriasis is the most common form [3, 4], and depending on the population studied, psoriatic arthritis (PsA) may occur in 5–42% of these patients [5]. Originally considered an epidermal keratinocyte dis-

KARGER

Fax +41 61 306 12 34
E-Mail karger@karger.ch
www.karger.com


1018–8665/10/2215–0043$26.00/0

Accessible online at:
www.karger.com/drm

Marina Papoutsaki, MD
Third Department of Dermatology
A. Sygros Hospital, Semitelou 6
GR–11528 Athens (Greece)
E-Mail marinapapoutsaki@hotmail.com

order, psoriasis has been proven to be one of the most common immune-mediated diseases, and numerous studies have suggested that proinflammatory cytokines, in particular tumour necrosis factor (TNF), serve a key role in potentiating inflammatory responses associated with both psoriasis and PsA [6–11].

Advances in the understanding of the immunopathogenesis of psoriasis and PsA have led to the introduction of biologic therapies [12]. Infliximab, a monoclonal antibody that binds with high affinity and specificity to TNF, has received approval for the treatment of plaque-type psoriasis and PsA. Other biologic therapies for the treatment of plaque-type psoriasis include etanercept, adalimumab and ustekinumab. Placebo-controlled studies and comparative randomised studies have shown that these agents produce a rapid and sustained response in psoriasis patients [13–18]. However, these studies provide data limited to one year of treatment; taking into consideration the chronic and recurrent nature of psoriasis, information on longer-term outcomes is needed. The methodology used to analyse data from short-term studies may not be appropriate to use when analysing data from long-term studies [19]. One of the major challenges in acquiring and analysing long-term data is loss to follow-up. During the course of a long-term study, patients may relocate and no longer be available for efficacy visits, or they may drop out of the study due to loss of efficacy or other reasons, such as adverse events or the initiation of a different treatment; these latter reasons may or may not be partially related to efficacy.

Various methods of analysis are used to account for missing assessments over long-term observations of biologic therapy efficacy. Non-responder imputation (NRI) is a relatively conservative approach to accounting for missing assessments in that this analysis considers subjects who have been lost to follow-up as non-responders. The observed values analysis essentially ignores subjects who have discontinued the study and includes only the values actually observed. The last observation carried forward (LOCF) approach is more liberal in that it assumes subjects who have been lost to follow-up are still responding based on the last observed data. The LOCF approach has been used in recent presentations of the long-term efficacy of adalimumab and etanercept [16, 20], while the NRI approach was used in the EXPRESS study of infliximab [14]. We conducted a retrospective analysis of 3 years of open-label infliximab use in patients affected by plaque-type psoriasis with or without PsA who were unresponsive, intolerant or had contraindications to conventional systemic agents. Using the data from this study, we explored the impact of selecting a particular analytical approach (NRI, observed values or LOCF) when working with missing data.

## Study Overview

One hundred and thirty-three patients (88 male, 45 female) with plaque-type psoriasis and a Psoriasis Area and Severity Index (PASI) score ranging from 0.1 to 61.2 (mean PASI score 14) were analysed. PsA was also present in 69 of these patients. Patients were between 25 and 81 years old (mean 49.1) and were unresponsive, intolerant or in certain cases, had contraindications (due to coexisting comorbidities) to conventional systemic treatments (methotrexate, ciclosporin, retinoids, psoralen plus ultraviolet A, fumaric acid esters). All patients gave written informed consent prior to treatment. The study protocol conformed to the ethical guidelines of the Declaration of Helsinki.

Infliximab was administered intravenously at 5 mg/kg at weeks 0, 2 and 6 (induction treatment), followed by treatment every 8 weeks. Efficacy was evaluated in all patients prior to each infusion at baseline, weeks 2 and 6 and then every 8 weeks by using the PASI score. Laboratory parameters were evaluated prior to the first infusion at baseline, at the end of induction and on a routine basis approximately every 6 months thereafter.

Of the 133 patients who initiated therapy, 2 (1.5%) interrupted treatment during the induction period: one due to lack of response and one due to loss to follow-up. Of the patients who completed induction (n = 131), 118 (90.7%) reached 6 months of treatment, while 13 stopped administration of the drug: 5 lost efficacy, one abandoned treatment because of an adverse event (acute renal failure after suffering from chronic renal insufficiency at inclusion) and 7 were included in other experimental protocols while still being PASI 75 responders. A total of 87 patients (73.7%) reached 1 year of therapy, and 31 discontinued infliximab. In particular, 7 patients stopped treatment because of loss of efficacy, one experienced an adverse event (myocardial infarction), one was lost to follow-up, 14 were included in other experimental protocols while still being PASI 75 responders and 8 stopped therapy due to reimbursement issues. Among the 87 patients who concluded 1 year of treatment, 44 (50.6%) reached 2 years of therapy and 43 discontinued therapy: 19 lost efficacy, 2 experienced adverse events (laryngeal dysplasia, severe dyspnoea), 11 were included in other experimental protocols while still being PASI 75 responders, 11 continued their treatment in other centres and one was lost to follow-up. Among the 43 patients who concluded 2 years of treatment, 32 (74.4%) reached 3 years of therapy. Of 10 patients who discontinued treatment between years 2 and 3, one lost efficacy and 9 continued their treatment in other centres.

As described, we approached missing PASI values due to infliximab discontinuation or loss to follow-up over 3 years at our clinic in three ways: (1) we imputed the last observed PASI value over the remainder of the 3 years (LOCF approach), (2) we analysed observed values of continuing patients only (observed values analysis), and (3) we counted the patient as a non-responder if the patient discontinued infliximab due to loss of response, whereas we carried the last response forward if the patient discontinued treatment due to other reasons (modified NRI approach). A substantial number of patients discontinued infliximab to start other experimental protocols while still demonstrating a PASI 75 response, which justified the modification of the NRI approach.

### Results by Analysis Method

*Last Observation Carried Forward.* In our main analysis, the LOCF analysis, at week 6, 91.6% (n = 120) of patients achieved PASI 50, 72.5% (n = 95) achieved PASI 75 and 49.6% (n = 65) achieved PASI 90 (table 1). Efficacy continued to improve through week 24, with 89.3% (n = 117) of patients achieving PASI 50, 79.3% (n = 104) achieving PASI 75 and 70.2% (n = 92) achieving PASI 90. After 1 year of treatment, 81.7, 67.2 and 52.7% of patients maintained a PASI 50, PASI 75 and PASI 90 response, respectively. The efficacy of infliximab was maintained over 3 years of continuous infliximab treatment.

*Observed Values Analysis.* Data from the observed values (as-treated) analysis are presented in table 2. At week 6, 91.6% (n = 120), 71.7% (n = 94) and 48.1% (n = 63) of patients achieved PASI 50, PASI 75 and PASI 90, respectively. A PASI 75 response was observed in 81.4% (n = 96), 69% (n = 60), 76.2% (n = 32) and 75% (n = 24) of patients at week 24, 1 year, 2 years and 3 years, respectively.

*Non-Responder Imputation.* When patients who discontinued infliximab due to loss of efficacy were counted as non-responders, the PASI 75 response was 72.5% at week 6, 75.6% at week 24, 58% at 1 year, 44.3% at 2 years and 41.2% at 3 years (table 3).

To graphically illustrate the differences in efficacy that are seen when these three analyses are used, the percentages of patients achieving a PASI 75 response over 3 years based on the LOCF, observed values and modified NRI analyses have been plotted together in figure 1.

**Table 1.** LOCF analysis: percentage of patients achieving PASI 50, PASI 75 and PASI 90 at different time points (week 6 through 3 years)

| | Week 6 | Week 24 | 1 year | 2 years | 3 years |
|---|---|---|---|---|---|
| PASI 50 | 91.6% | 89.3% | 81.7% | 78.6% | 77.9% |
| Number in data set | 120 | 117 | 107 | 103 | 102 |
| PASI 75 | 72.5% | 79.3% | 67.2% | 67.9% | 65.6% |
| Number in data set | 95 | 104 | 88 | 89 | 86 |
| PASI 90 | 49.6% | 70.2% | 52.7% | 51.1% | 52.7% |
| Number in data set | 65 | 92 | 69 | 67 | 69 |

Denominator in each cell = 131.

**Table 2.** Observed values analysis: percentage of patients (as treated) achieving PASI 50, PASI 75 and PASI 90 at different time points (week 6 through 3 years)

| | Week 6 | Week 24 | 1 year | 2 years | 3 years |
|---|---|---|---|---|---|
| PASI 50 | 91.6% | 90.7% | 85.1% | 85.7% | 91.6% |
| n/N | 120/131 | 107/118 | 74/87 | 36/42 | 29/32 |
| PASI 75 | 71.7% | 81.4% | 69.0% | 76.2% | 75.0% |
| n/N | 94/131 | 96/118 | 60/87 | 32/42 | 24/32 |
| PASI 90 | 48.1% | 72.9% | 55.1% | 57.1% | 59.4% |
| n/N | 63/131 | 86/118 | 48/87 | 24/42 | 19/32 |

**Table 3.** Modified NRI analysis: percentage of patients achieving PASI 50, PASI 75 and PASI 90 at different time points (week 6 through 3 years)

| | Week 6 | Week 24 | 1 year | 2 years | 3 years |
|---|---|---|---|---|---|
| PASI 50 | 91.6% | 85.5% | 72.5% | 55.0% | 53.4% |
| Number in data set | 120 | 112 | 95 | 72 | 70 |
| PASI 75 | 72.5% | 75.6% | 58.0% | 44.3% | 41.2% |
| Number in data set | 95 | 99 | 76 | 58 | 54 |
| PASI 90 | 49.6% | 66.4% | 43.5% | 27.5% | 28.2% |
| Number in data set | 65 | 87 | 57 | 36 | 37 |

Denominator in each cell = 131; non-responder imputation for subjects who discontinued due to loss of efficacy; last observed values were used for other subjects lost to follow-up.

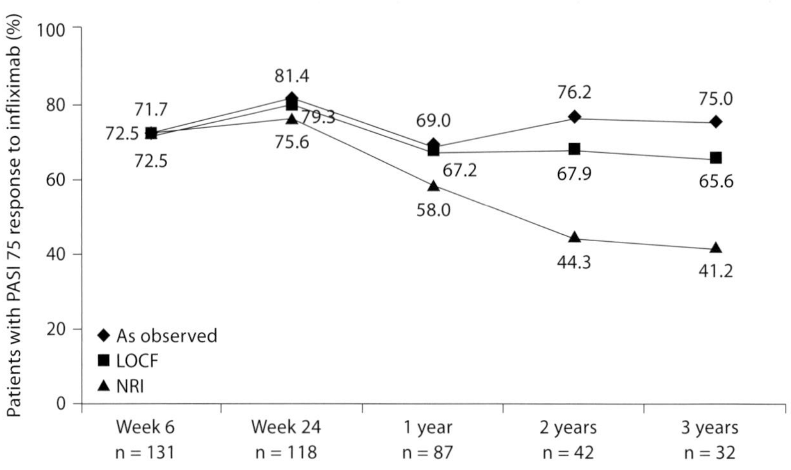


**Fig. 1.** Percentage of patients achieving PASI 75 while receiving infliximab over 3 years, plotted by LOCF, observed values and NRI analyses. LOCF = Last observation carried forward; NRI = non-responder imputation.

## Conclusions

The long-term treatment of patients affected by severe psoriasis may represent an important therapeutic challenge. Our data demonstrated that infliximab was effective in patients with plaque-type psoriasis by as early as week 6. This level of efficacy is comparable with that reported in the three randomised, placebo-controlled trials examining the efficacy of infliximab in moderate-to-severe, stable chronic plaque-type psoriasis [13–15] and a prospective, open-label study [21]. Our data also demonstrated the ability of infliximab to maintain this level of efficacy through 3 years. However, the most striking finding was that the estimate of the 3-year efficacy of infliximab varied from 41% with the NRI approach to 66% with the LOCF approach and 75% with the observed values approach. The efficacy almost doubled, depending on which analysis method was used to account for missing values.

Loss to follow-up is a major challenge in studies of long-term efficacy. After 3 years, we had observations on 32 of the 131 patients who initially started treatment – not an unusual rate in long-term observational studies. Various missing values strategies are used to deal with loss to follow-up of patients. In some long-term studies, only the observed data are reported, and patients whose follow-up is not available are not counted [19]. Some of these patients are no longer receiving treatment because of loss of efficacy, and we ignore this valuable information in observed values analyses. The data in table 2 demonstrate the result using this approach – a very high PASI response for infliximab.

An alternative strategy is to take the last observed value and carry this forward to subsequent time points, as was done in the open-label extension studies of adalimumab and etanercept [16, 20]. Our main analysis in table 1 represents this strategy. In this approach, we still counted 131 patients at the end of 3 years, even though a considerable proportion were no longer receiving the treatment, sometimes even after only 2 years. This illustrates the problem with a LOCF approach. However, since this approach is consistent with what has been reported for other agents, we considered this our main analysis. In our third approach, we carried forward all non-responders to subsequent time points, as was performed in the EXPRESS controlled study of infliximab [14], even when these patients might have regained a response at a later time. The juxtaposition of these three approaches clearly demonstrates the impact of the choice of a particular missing values strategy on the results of long-term efficacy studies. In its technical guidance for clinical trials, the International Conference on Harmonisation of Technical Requirements for Registration of Pharmaceuticals for Human Use (ICH; the body that sets standards for the requirements for registration of pharmaceutical products) notes that various techniques are available to deal with missing values and recommends that an investigation be made concerning the sensitivity of the results of an analysis to the method of handling missing data [22]. We demonstrated that when observed values or LOCF approaches are used, the results of the more conservative NRI approach should be presented as well to give a fair overview of the long-term efficacy of a treatment for plaque-type psoriasis.

## Conflicts of Interest

M. Papoutsaki has served as a consultant for Schering-Plough and as a speaker for Schering Corporation, a subsidiary of Merck & Co., Inc. and Abbott. A. Costanzo has served as a speaker for Serono. S. Chimenti has served as a consultant and speaker for Wyeth, Centocor and Schering Corporation.

## References


1 Griffiths CEM, Barker J: Pathogenesis and clinical features of psoriasis. Lancet 2007; 370:263–271.
2 Christophers E: Psoriasis – epidemiology and clinical spectrum. Clin Exp Dermatol 2001;26:314–320.
3 Lebwohl M: Psoriasis. Lancet 2003;361: 1197–1204.
4 Schon MP, Boehncke WH: Psoriasis. N Engl J Med 2005;352:1899–1912.
5 Gladman DD, Brockbank J: Psoriatic arthritis. Expert Opin Investig Drugs 2000;9:1511–1522.
6 Ettehadi P, Greaves MW, Wallach D, Aderka D, Camp RD: Elevated tumor necrosis factor-α (TNFα) biological activity in psoriatic skin lesions. Clin Exp Immunol 1994;96: 146–151.
7 Höhler T, Kruger A, Schneider PM, Schopf RE, Knop J, Rittner C, Meyer zum Büschenfelde KH, Märker-Hermann E: A TNF-α promoter polymorphism is associated with juvenile onset of psoriasis and psoriatic arthritis. J Invest Dermatol 1997;109:562–565.
8 Partsch G, Steiner G, Leeb BF, Dunky A, Bröll H, Smolen JS: Highly increased levels of tumor necrosis factor-α and other proinflammatory cytokines in psoriatic arthritis synovial fluid. J Rheumatol 1997;24:518–523.
9 Ritchlin C, Haas-Smith SA, Hicks D, Cappuccio J, Osterland CK, Looney RJ: Patterns of cytokine production in psoriatic synovium. J Rheumatol 1998;25:1544–1552.
10 Danning CL, Illei GG, Hitchon C, Greer MR, Boumpas DT, McInnes IB: Macrophage-derived cytokine and nuclear factor κB p65 expression in synovial membrane and skin of patients with psoriatic arthritis. Arthritis Rheum 2000;43:1244–1256.
11 Partsch G, Wagner E, Leeb BF, Dunky A, Steiner G, Smolen JS: Upregulation of cytokine receptors sTNF-R55, sTNF-R75, and sIL-2R in psoriatic arthritis synovial fluid. J Rheumatol 1998;25:105–110.
12 Boss JD, de Rie MA: The pathogenesis of psoriasis: immunological facts and speculations. Immunol Today 1999;20:40–46.
13 Gottlieb AB, Evans R, Li S, Dooley LT, Guzzo CA, Baker D, Bala M, Marano CW, Menter A: Infliximab induction therapy for patients with severe plaque-type psoriasis: a randomized, double-blind, placebo-controlled trial. J Am Acad Dermatol 2004;51:534–542.
14 Reich K, Nestle FO, Papp K, Ortonne JP, Evans R, Guzzo C, Li S, Dooley LT, Griffiths CE: Infliximab induction and maintenance therapy for moderate-to-severe psoriasis: a phase III, multicentre, double-blind trial. Lancet 2005;366:1367–1374.
15 Menter A, Feldman SR, Weinstein GD, Papp K, Evans R, Guzzo C, Li S, Dooley LT, Arnold C, Gottlieb AB: A randomized comparison of continuous vs. intermittent infliximab maintenance regimens over 1 year in the treatment of moderate-to-severe plaque psoriasis. J Am Acad Dermatol 2007;56:1–15.
16 Tyring S, Gordon KB, Poulin Y, Langley RG, Gottlieb AB, Dunn M, Jahreis A: Long-term safety and efficacy of 50 mg of etanercept twice weekly in patients with psoriasis. Arch Dermatol 2007;143:719–726.
17 Menter A, Tyring SK, Gordon K, Kimball AB, Leonardi CL, Langley RG, Strober BE, Kaul M, Gu Y, Okun M, Papp K: Adalimumab therapy for moderate to severe psoriasis: a randomized, controlled phase III trial. J Am Acad Dermatol 2008;58:106–115.
18 Papp KA, Langley RG, Lebwohl M, Krueger GG, Szapary P, Yeilding N, Guzzo C, Hsu MC, Wang Y, Li S, Dooley LT, Reich K; PHOENIX 2 study investigators: Efficacy and safety of ustekinumab, a human interleukin-12/23 monoclonal antibody, in patients with psoriasis: 52-week results from a randomised, double-blind, placebo-controlled trial (PHOENIX 2). Lancet 2008;371: 1675–1684.
19 Papp KA, Fonjallaz P, Casset-Semanaz F, Krueger JG, Wittkowski KM: Analytical approaches to reporting long-term clinical trial data. Curr Med Res Opin 2008;24:2001–2008.
20 Gordon KB, Tyring S, Gu Y, Okun MM: Psoriasis patients treated continuously with adalimumab: efficacy and safety results from months 12 to 18 (abstract). J Am Acad Dermatol 2008;58:AB129 (abstract P2654).
21 Smith CH, Jackson K, Bashir SJ, Perez A, Chew AL, Powell AM, Wain M, Barker JN: Infliximab for severe, treatment-resistant psoriasis: a prospective, open-label study. Br J Dermatol 2006;155:160–169.
22 ICH Expert Working Group: ICH harmonised tripartite guideline. Statistical principles for clinical trials. 5 February 1998.

Dermatology

## Author Index Vol. 221, Suppl. 1, 2010



## Subject Index Vol. 221, Suppl. 1, 2010



KARGER

Fax +41 61 306 12 34
E-Mail karger@karger.ch
www.karger.com



Accessible online at:
www.karger.com/drm